Our
Endangered
Hearing

Our Endangered Hearing

Understanding & Coping with Hearing Loss

By Richard Carmen

Rodale Press Emmaus, PA

Copyright © 1977 Rodale Press, Inc.

Library of Congress Cataloging in Publication Data
Carmen, Richard.
  Our endangered hearing.

  Includes index.
  1. Hearing disorders. I. Title.
RF290.C37   617.8'9   76-58359
ISBN 0-87857-165-5

Printed on recycled paper

2 4 6 8 10 9 7 5 3

To Loren

Acknowledgments

I wish to express the gratitude I have for my family, and their support, encouragement and agreement during the many months of writing this book.

In preparation of the manuscript, I am indebted to several people for their encouragement, active participation, and review of the material. I especially appreciate the contributions from Joel Hurvitz, M.A., Audiologist, Los Angeles Ear Medical Group; Dion Svihovec, Ph.D., Audiologist, Veterans Administration Hospital, Sepulveda, California; and Bettye W. Smith, Ph.D., Chief of Audiology and Speech Pathology Services, Veterans Administration Outpatient Clinic, Los Angeles, California. Through a willingness to share and the ability to communicate, they have been extremely helpful in the development of ideas, material and direction that I feel have been for the betterment of this book. Their kindnesses as friends and critiques as colleagues will long be remembered.

I am grateful to the physicians in the Ear, Nose and Throat Clinic of the Southern California Permanente Medical Group in Panorama City, California, for having afforded me an opportunity to become actively involved in the clinical aspects of audiology. I also express my appreciation to all the competent women in the clinic who keep things running efficiently. Many of the people in this clinic have been a very important part of my life.

There are many people who I would truly like to acknowledge as having had a positive effect on my professional life and therefore on this book. Somehow, it wouldn't be practical to name them all.

I sincerely thank Patsy for her superb typing (and her patience in re-typing my sudden changes). And I thank Annie C. for her ingenuity and love.

Table of Contents

Preface

I have written this book for the benefit of hearing impaired individuals as well as for those people who desire to learn about this sensory deprivation and may not suffer from a loss of hearing at all.

There presently is no source of information available for hearing impaired people to turn to other than inadequate brochures or technical books written for professionals in audiology.

From my experience, I have found that many people hold onto beliefs about hearing loss that are often based on rumor. I have tried to clarify much of this misinformation by explaining what it means to hear as well as what it means to lose your hearing.

In addition to discussing the causes of and treatments for hearing loss, I have discussed what can be done to prevent hearing loss. It is apparent that noise is the greatest enemy of the ears. Abatement of noise will mean longer years of hearing for everybody.

My discussion of hearing aids, as well as the questions and answers about them, should dispel the many misconceptions regarding aids. The purchase of a hearing aid is usually the start of handling a hearing problem, but it is seldom the solution. Many people cling to unrealistic expectations about hearing aids that can lead to quite a letdown, complicating the hearing problem with depression.

Counseling by an audiologist is the most important link—and all too often the greatest missing link—between wanting to resolve a hearing problem and finally taking action to resolve the problem. But unfortunately, hearing health professionals (including me) cannot possibly afford the time that it takes to inform each patient of their particular hearing problem.

Therefore, while my ultimate goal in this book is to encourage you who have a hearing loss to better understand this sensory deprivation and to provide a way for others to prevent hearing loss, I also hope that this book will facilitate the needed counseling by other professionals for their patients.

Hippocrates has said: HEALING IS A MATTER OF TIME BUT IT IS ALSO A MATTER OF OPPORTUNITY.

r.c.

Chapter I
THE SILENT HANDICAP

Hearing is one of our most valued senses. We depend on it for most of our communication and to orient ourselves in our environment. A decreased sensitivity in hearing would limit many daily functions that are often taken for granted. But impaired hearing does not stop at just deficient hearing. It influences nearly every aspect of our lives. Learning becomes more difficult—so does maintaining employment. Lasting friendships are harder to make and keep. Mixed feelings of isolation, embarrassment and frustration can lead to anxiety or despair. Confidence and security may dwindle, and we may feel our very existence threatened.

Though most of us take normal hearing for granted, the odds are stacked against us all. There is *one* chance in *ten* that you will have *normal* hearing by age 65. But we are the creatures who created these odds. We have created the primary element responsible for these unfortunate consequences—NOISE. Hearing loss is not caused by noise alone, though it is certainly the number one cause. Negligence with ear infections can produce permanent hearing loss. Strong and compelling evidence exists that diet affects hearing. The drugs we take can affect our hearing, and even hearing aids can decrease hearing if improperly fitted.

SOUND FACTS

Traditionally, estimates of how many people suffer from a hearing loss have been unrealistically low. My own calculations show that about 15 percent of the present population in the United States (over 33 million people) have a significant hearing impairment.

We know that of the 75 million industrial workers in the United States, a very rock bottom minimum estimate of 25 percent presently have a hearing loss that prevents effective communication. This means that 18,750,000 people employed in industry have impaired hearing. This does not mean that they are all *directly* exposed to dangerous noise levels. They are not. But *indirect* exposure that secretaries, accountants and other office personnel get is enough to produce serious hearing impairment—*and it does!*

The United States Occupational Safety and Health Administration (OSHA) reported in 1975 that based on a survey of 19 major industries, an estimated 36 percent of production workers are likely to suffer hearing losses attributable to noise *before the age of sixty.* I have used a more conservative statistic.

In addition to the industrial workers, there are more than 21 million Americans over the age of 65 at this time. Approximately 28 percent of this population suffer from serious communicative problems due directly to a serious loss of hearing. Therefore, at least 5,880,000 senior citizens experience real hearing problems. But we also know that 88 percent of those age 65 and older have *some degree* of hearing loss. Exactly what is and what is not a serious communicative disorder as a result of hearing loss is extremely difficult to determine. It is my own opinion that probably 50 percent or more have such a serious hearing handicap.

We know that approximately 10 percent of the 30 million children in public schools in the United States have impaired hearing at this very moment. Many of these school children (mostly male) have permanent high frequency hearing loss due to their exposure to cap guns, air rifles, firecrackers, carpentry, excessively loud music, etc. This results in three million young children with impaired hearing that can be statistically accounted for. However, there are approximately 20 million more children under the age of 18 who are not enrolled in public schools. If 10 percent of this group also experience a hearing loss (and indeed there is every reason why this group should), then another two million children under 18 have impaired hearing.

The majority of children suffer from fluid in the ears which can result in a permanent loss of hearing if left untreated.[1] Also, researchers still don't know the cause of hearing loss in 20 to 40 percent of all children with congenital hearing deficiencies.[2] The number of children affected may well increase if the cause is not discovered.

There are an estimated 1,800,000 deaf people in the United States. There are also people with impaired hearing who cannot be categorized as industrial workers, are not over age 65, are not children under 18 and are not deaf. This remaining population consists of approximately 100 million Americans for whom no estimate has been made yet. The American Speech and Hearing Association has reported that approximately 10 percent of the population has some degree of hearing loss. But I differ with their calculations. Only a matter of a few years ago they were reporting many millions less than they are presently. This is because their accuracy has increased. But for the sake of argument, I will calculate two and one-half percent (instead of 10 percent) for the remaining 100 million people that do not fit into any category thus far mentioned. In so doing, I am estimating that this remaining group has a serious communicative problem directly due to hearing impairment. Thus, at least 2,500,000 more people have a serious hearing deficit.

This amounts to a lot of people with loss of hearing:

18,750,000 industrial workers now with impaired hearing
 5,880,000 people over the age of 65 with impaired hearing
 5,000,000 children under age 18 with impaired hearing
 1,800,000 deaf persons
 2,500,000 people in the remaining population with impaired hearing

----

33,930,000 people with seriously impaired hearing in the United States

AND HEARING LOSS IS ON THE INCREASE!

The need to change the current trend is apparent. The United States Public Health Service has announced that impaired hearing is now the nation's greatest handicapping condition, affecting more people than any other chronic ailment. In pure numbers alone, there are more people with hearing impairments than the total population of Arizona, Arkansas, Colorado, Delaware, Hawaii, Idaho, Iowa, Kansas, Maine, Mississippi, Montana, Nebraska, Nevada, New Hampshire, New Mexico, North Dakota, South Dakota, Rhode Island, Utah, West Virginia and Wyoming COMBINED!!

Surveys have revealed that it takes the average hearing impaired individual five years before receiving treatment for the condition.[3] In that five-year interim, the problem could easily worsen.

Hearing loss can occur at any age, in any degree, to either sex and apart from any other physical anomaly. How others react to a hearing loss is often as much of a problem as the loss itself. Discrimination against people with hearing difficulties still exists. The hearing impaired suffer from some of the same social stigmas and emotional turmoil today as they did hundreds of years ago. They are frequently the targets of ridicule and the victims of embarrassment, shame and isolation. Because of such social oppression, people with hearing difficulties tend to keep the affliction secret. As a result, there may be many more people afflicted with hearing impairment than statistically indicated.

SOUND MYTHS

There have been as many myths associated with hearing loss as there are people to talk about it: stupidity, senility, mental deficiency, cripplement, old age, slowness, inability to speak or function normally, and on and on. These descriptions were widely believed up through the 19th century. We are seemingly more civilized in the 20th century but we are still greatly impatient with hard of hearing individuals and lack much insight into the true nature of this communicative disorder.

The greatest inaccuracy down through history has been the use of the word "dumb." We all have heard the expression "deaf and dumb" but this is no reference to intelligence. "Deaf" is self-explanatory. But "dumb" refers to an inability to speak or use the speech organs to communicate. It is an unfortunate choice for a word to describe such an infirmity and the fact that the word is still a part of many people's vocabulary only reinforces the myths that surely must go with it.

THE EFFECTS OF HEARING LOSS

Extensive research has been carried out in the area of hearing loss and its effects on the many aspects of human development. This research, unfortunately, has been primarily a study of those people afflicted with very severe or profound hearing loss (deafness) and therefore any generalizations made about this group or about deafness must be made with great caution as it is applied to hard of hearing people.

I am primarily concerned with a partial loss of hearing because there is so plainly a lack of material available to inform professionals and hearing impaired people about what the affliction can do to change attitude, ideas, direction in life, relationships, etc. The deaf as a population have been far easier to study and evaluate than hard of hearing groups. Deaf children are usually in schools for the deaf while hard of hearing children are quite frequently integrated into schools for the hearing. Their study is therefore more difficult. Hard of hearing adults are even more difficult to evaluate because so many ignore the problem, often waiting for it to get "bad enough" before they choose to do something about it. We are only recently coming to realize that even a partial loss of hearing can have serious effects on one's life, the most significant effect being a feeling of separation.

The effects that any handicap will have on us are largely determined by the age at which it appears and the degree of the impairment itself. Also, to better understand the effects of

5

hearing loss, we must be fully aware of how important hearing really is.

CHILDREN

We know that children deaf from birth experience a tremendous language deficit. It is difficult to build a language that is based upon spoken words when those spoken words cannot be heard. Although the deaf can use sign language to communicate (manually), sign language is a very limited system, with many possible concepts represented by one sign, and no sign for other concepts that need clarification. Verbal languages as we know them contain hundreds of thousands of words and we generally can find the word we need to represent the concept we desire to communicate. Not being able to find the word that represents what we want to say creates a great deal of frustration. Also, if one is taught *only* sign language, one *thinks* only in sign language. And since language that is manual is a greatly limiting language, it represents a limited number of ideas, thereby limiting the potential of mental development for many deaf people. Research bears this out.

Deafness does influence intelligence through a language handicap. Deaf children have greater difficulty with abstraction than hearing children. Research indicates evidence of poorer retention and recall (memory) abilities among deaf persons than hearing children. As would be expected, when deaf children have been tested on their verbal ability as compared to normal hearing children, they scored rather consistently below average. This data cannot be applied to all deaf people. However, the lack of language development, be it caused by deafness or some other affliction, can adversely affect the mental development of any human being.

Language as we know it is learned primarily through our sensory channel of hearing. When we learn new words by hearing them frequently enough in conversation, we slowly incorporate these new words into our own language. When these new words are not learned because of a hearing impairment, then a language impairment may result.

Since reading ability depends upon language (receiving

words that represent thoughts and ideas and understanding them), if a language handicap is present, a reading handicap is also likely. A survey by Gallaudet College in 1971 revealed that by age 19, many deaf and hard of hearing children had reading competence levels equivalent to less than 5th grade.

When hearing loss prevents the reception of words, not only language becomes limited, but so do other areas, as we will see.

We must keep in mind that children, like adults, monitor their world by what they see and hear. The normal functions of sight and sound are critical in an infant's development if he is to become a well-adjusted adult. Vision and audition help an infant to feel as though he is a part of the world, regardless of his ability to participate in this world. Lack of sight or sound breaks off this sense of belonging. It creates a feeling of separateness in an infant, as well as in an adult. The implications of a hearing impairment during infancy, even if mild, are alarming.

A hearing loss of 30 to 40 decibels (dB) in an infant, a loss considered by professionals to be "mild," can produce a 15 to 20 percent reduction in vocabulary development. Such a reduction at such an early age can have a serious and permanent effect upon the child—including reading, language, social maturity and above all, mental development. The longer that the hearing loss remains with a growing child, particularly within the first two years of development, the greater the risk of developmental problems.

We know that as normal hearing children mature, they become more independent and more socially competent (and confident). Studies reveal that this is also true for hard of hearing persons. But deaf individuals become less socially mature each year and reveal greater dependence on other people than normal or hard of hearing persons. It is this dependence that becomes the real handicap. I will discuss "handicap" in more detail later in this chapter.

The particular relationship that social maturity has to emotional and educational development deserves mentioning. There is a positive correlation between the degree of social

7

maturity and the level of emotional adjustment and educational achievements. Research supports the idea that the more socially competent one is, the greater the emotional and educational development. And we may assume that speech and hearing are the fundamental channels through which such competence is achieved. We cannot make great strides in formal education when education is based on language and language is based on being able to speak and hear.

The later in life that hearing loss occurs, the less the psychological effect. Infants deaf from birth are far more isolated from the world that surrounds them than the infants who develop hearing impairments later, after they have recognized that there is a world out there. Our ability to hear the world and see the world helps us to establish and maintain contact with the realities of that world. Early deprivation of hearing can also create a deprivation of sensory contact with our environment.

Emotional development is less affected when hearing loss develops in later school years, because with age, one becomes more emotionally adjusted. We can be more understanding of the problem of a hearing deficit as we grow older and in so doing, become more tolerant. An infant never gets this opportunity. Nevertheless, even in school years, a hearing loss is not easy to deal with. Though a school age child is older and more emotionally mature than an infant, it is not easy for a child to face a hearing problem. Social relationships are very often seriously affected as a result of impaired communication. The older we get, the greater the social impact of hearing loss on our lives.

ADULTS

If hearing loss occurs between the ages of 18 and 30, although the psychological effects are present, the social effects are tremendous. Early school years make for the development of nice and close relationships—but not the kind of relationships that are created and depended upon when we are over 18. Relationships are taken more seriously and therefore, the loss of relationships are taken equally more seriously. Profound psychosocial effects are visible in hard of hearing persons in many aspects of their lives. This includes marital problems, changing friends and acquaintances, and changing personal directions and goals, as with a change in employment or move out of a city.

When hearing loss occurs in more mature adults, particularly over the age of 30, occupation is affected most, with social relationships not quite as seriously affected. Since the basic personality develops at a very young age, the psychological effects are greatest in children.

We cannot forget the importance of the degree of a hearing impairment. Regardless of age, the greater the hearing loss, the greater are the psychological effects.

PSYCHOLOGICAL EFFECTS AND PERSONALITY

Research into the area of hearing loss and its effects on personality have revealed much about the problems created by this sensory deprivation. It is interesting to note one researcher reporting that a group of deaf individuals did not consider their problem a handicap, yet hard of hearing individuals did.[4] This is attributed to the fact that the hard of hearing group once possessed normal hearing and were therefore more aware of what they had lost.

All of us have extrovert or introvert traits. No one is a "pure" introvert or extrovert, but one of the traits is usually dominant in each of us.

A person's ability to handle a hearing impairment (or for that matter, any handicap) can often be determined through personality. The more extroverted a person is, the greater the chances of adjustment. Positive thinkers adjust more quickly than depressed or negative thinkers. The extroverted individual who develops a hearing impairment finds that by his very nature alone, he is more capable of handling the problem (perhaps because he does more talking than listening). "Withdrawn," "isolated," or "lonely" are more descriptive of an introvert than an extrovert. But even an extroverted individual may find himself in isolation if he does not resolve his problem.

9

Since isolation is not a fundamental part of an extrovert, he may seek all kinds of help to keep from becoming isolated.

The more introverted hard of hearing person finds himself generally comfortable with such descriptions as "reserved," "quiet," or "inward." Many introverts are withdrawn, isolated and lonely. This group is the target of the greatest torment, much of it self-inflicted. They may not particularly mind solitude and may appreciate silence. They are the most difficult people to inspire to resolve their handicap because the mere presence of their handicap only reinforces their basic nature. Withdrawal can be as easily equated with introversion as it can be with the end result of a long-standing hearing loss. Introverts may look forward to seclusion. Hearing loss may drive a person to seclusion. They often can be one and the same, thereby allowing such a person to suffer much longer than necessary with the impairment.

By and large, the more introverted person is more hassled by other people recommending that he get help than by the hearing loss itself. Family and friends are often more bothered than the victim. Although there is a level of frustration that will build up in anyone when effective communication is no longer possible, an introvert is often too tolerant of the problem and will not usually seek help alone. It might take the encouragement of a friend, a niece, a grandson or a mother.

HEARING LOSS IN THE ELDERLY

With the added factor of age, isolation can be deadly. Old age is a lonely period for most people—a time when company is so meaningful and communication so necessary. Among the more than 21 million Americans presently over the age of 65, the vast majority have been excommunicated in one way or another by family, friends or society.

Even normal hearing senior citizens suffer from isolation, but a hearing loss only intensifies these feelings. Early in the 1970's, the United States National Health Survey in geriatrics reported that 13 to 25 percent of those age 65 and older were affected by hearing loss. By 1975, the Senate Congressional Record stated that at least 88 percent of all Americans age 65 and older experienced *some* degree of hearing loss. This was clarified by the American Speech and Hearing Association in 1976 when they reported that at least 28 percent of all Americans age 65 and older experienced *serious communicative disorders* due to hearing loss. If we use the 28 percent figure, then nearly six million people over the age of 65 suffer from serious communicative disorders as a result of hearing loss. One study showed that 90 percent of all people living in nursing homes suffer from serious hearing disorders. The rate of hearing loss increases among the elderly by 250,000 people each year (see "Presbycusis," p. 50).

INVISIBLE DAMAGE

Sympathy we have for the blind man who walks with a red-tipped cane. But hearing loss is not an obvious condition. Disease of the middle or inner ear is an internal problem only recognizable to a stranger through aural communication. "Why the hell don't you listen to what I'm telling you? Do I have to repeat myself again?", "What's the matter with you, any-way? . . . Oh . . . Oh, you have a hearing loss. I didn't know that."

Certainly the burden of hearing loss could be shared through an understanding of difficulties that the normal hearing person doesn't experience in listening. Running with two broken legs is not easy. Somebody may ask you to run, but it must be explained that a physical situation can't allow it. Hearing loss is a physical condition, not nearly as apparent as a broken leg. On a one-to-one conversational level, if the speaker would only slow the speech down a bit and not run so fast, if he would only speak more distinctly rather than tripping over words, a hearing loss may not be so impairing when com-municating.

FRAGMENTED HEARING AND ENTANGLED EMOTIONS

One of the first emotions that a hearing deficient person goes through is embarrassment. It becomes too disconcerting to constantly request statements to be repeated. You either hear the words or try to assemble fragments of speech into something meaningful. This involves guesswork and the odds are against successful assemblage of fragmented words. Frequently, somebody with a hearing loss may give a totally inappropriate response to a question. For example, a person with a moderate high frequency hearing loss (making consonant sounds difficult to hear) may walk into the kitchen where his wife is preparing homemade cookies for her club luncheon that afternoon. She may ask her husband to sit down, "Have a seat." In the meantime, he hears the sounds of these words as "Have a piece" and reaches into the platter of neatly placed cookies where his hand meets the force of a plummeting spatula. Both parties may never realize what took place unless the husband comes back with "Well, I thought you said have a piece!" or the wife shouts "Get away from these—they're for the ladies today!" The husband could be greatly confused by his wife offering a cookie to him and then striking him for taking it. On the other hand, a woman could be greatly confused by her husband's apparent lack of concern for her baking by grabbing a cookie. All of this because of a hearing problem which both pass off as a "misunderstanding."

Many choose to ignore or hide their hearing deficiency, which only results in mounting frustration. Everyone may laugh at a joke, but you may have missed the punchline. Do you ask to have it repeated or do you laugh with the rest of the group? If you have no problem with hearing, you most likely would ask to have it repeated. But if you suffer from a hearing impairment, you may well hesitate to ask for statements to be repeated. Often it can be much less frustrating and less embarrassing to go along with the group and laugh than to risk feeling uncomfortable by having it repeated.

Such situations can soon become threatening for hearing impaired persons. People should be aware of the hearing difficulty so that inappropriate responses are not misconstrued. Giving a wrong answer to a question can produce unnecessary humiliation unless the problem is opened-up instead of covered-up.

Frustration can lead to depression if it goes unchecked. It

may be a fast road from "Well, I'll try to hear" to "I'm afraid to hear." Anxiety may take over, leading to discouragement and fatigue. Disappointment reinforced by a continual inability to hear properly can create withdrawal (i.e., from threatening situations of communication). And withdrawal may ultimately lead to isolation. For some, isolation may mean more reading, writing, creative or artistic endeavors, but unfortunately hearing impaired people do not enjoy the type of isolation they are forced into. It is a lonely world. It's a place most would rather escape from than escape to. They may possess deep feelings of rejection or hostility. A human being once so gentle, thoughtful, kind and understanding may be trapped within himself, unable and/or unwilling to come out. Despair is often the outcome.

Ludwig van Beethoven is one of history's most outstanding examples of what hearing loss can do to the human spirit. At the age of 28, having already composed over 50 major pieces of music, he began to slowly lose his hearing. At the age of 32, Beethoven wrote a letter of suicide to his brothers. The letter was written in 1802, but not delivered because, in fact, he did not commit suicide:

How could I declare the weakness of a sense which in me ought to be more acute than in others—a sense which formerly I possessed in highest perfection, a perfection such as few in my profession enjoy, or ever have enjoyed . . . . Forgive me, therefore, if you see me withdraw, when I would willingly mix with you. My misfortune pains me doubly in that I am certain to be misunderstood. For me, there can be no recreation in the society of my fellow creatures, no refined conversations, no interchange of thought. Almost alone, and only mixing in society when absolutely necessary, I am compelled to live as an exile. If I approach near to people, a feeling of hot anxiety comes over me lest my condition should be noticed—for so it was during these past six months which I spent in the country. Ordered by my intelligent physician to spare my hearing as much as possible, he almost fell in with my present frame of mind, although many a time I was carried away by my sociable inclinations. But how humiliating was it, when someone standing close to me heard a distant flute, and I heard nothing, or a shepherd singing, and again I heard nothing. Such incidents almost drove me to despair; at times I was on the point of putting an end to my life. . . .[5]

Beethoven exemplifies the tragedy brought about by deprived hearing. His loss was very gradual and progressive. By the age of 48, Beethoven lost his hearing completely. Even so, he continued to write music although he could no longer hear it performed.

PREHISTORIC MAN, MODERN MAN AND HEARING

Early man, 100,000 years ago, depended upon his own ability to hunt to provide his family with food and clothing. Each family within a group or cluster of families was independent, responsible for taking care of themselves. There was little assistance from "friends." If the man or head of a family unit was unsuccessful in hunting, edibles that the women and children gathered were the primary sustenance. But families did not live for extended periods solely on fruits. Man was not a vegetarian, he was carnivorous. Animals provided meat for food, hides for clothing and bones for making tools and weapons. Hunting became a necessity—it meant survival. Once a man was proven to be an unsuccessful hunter, he was either abandoned or accepted as a weaker entity in the group, allowed to help women and children gather. A woman and her children were then forced to adopt another man into the clan capable of hunting. In an early society where "macho" or "machismo" meant strength enough to keep more than oneself alive, those incapable of providing were often found to be a burden. Their abandonment was sometimes a matter of necessity among nomads whose destinies were uncertain. Movement meant survival.

If for some reason a man was maimed, handicapped or incapable of hunting due to a mild or serious physical condition, he was automatically a liability, not an asset to a family. If a handicapped hunter was left alone, incapable of hunting or even keeping up with a group, he would die, unable to provide food and shelter for himself. If he was accepted into his own family as a gatherer, he was usually looked upon as a cast-away, weakling or failure, regardless of his ability to gather. Gathering was an established responsibility for women and children—not men. Such a set of circumstances could have been devastating to the ego of such a hunter.

Hence, "handicap" carried great implications even tens of thousands of years ago. A man could not hunt well if he could not hear well. Without audition, man was incapable of hearing the fine movements of his prey. He could not locate their feeding or nesting areas easily or inconspicuously. He depended upon his acute hearing for sounds that came from beyond his visual field. The extent of his handicap was often measured by the degree of his dependence upon others for his own survival. Certainly it could be said that of all early man's senses, audition and vision were most important for successful hunting. Injury to either was a potential deadly handicap.

As we approach the 21st century, our basic purpose is still survival. Technology has made many physical aspects of our lives much easier, but new obstacles now challenge us. Present-day man has created a complex society in which many new skills are needed for continued survival. Communication is primary among these skills. Since communication is far more sophisticated and complex today than even 10 years ago (let alone 100,000 years ago), our hearing and our sight have a more significant role in our daily lives. A handicap to either sense still presents a threat to our survival.

ORIENTATION

Sight and sound provide us with our orientation and give us a perspective on our environment. One element may be judged as far away because it can barely be seen. Another element may be interpreted as distant because of its faint audibility. Our senses allow us to monitor the activities in our environment and help us to feel comfortable.

Lack of light does not frighten the blind or visually impaired because they have grown accustomed to this condition. Their orientation is not disturbed if their hearing is intact.

When communicating, the cues for the blind are primarily auditory, such as the sound of a closing door followed by fading footsteps, or interpreting meaning from a hesitation in speech, a change in pitch or inflection of the voice. These are as meaningful as a smile or shrug of the shoulders to the individual with sight. However, lack of light is an immediate threat to any hard of hearing person, compounding the hearing impairment with a visual impairment as well.

If your orientation is upset, you are likely to go on the defensive: "Is the telephone ringing?", "Did the dishwasher turn off?", "Did . . .?" Relaxation becomes impossible if you do not feel secure in your environment. None of us can see around corners, but we may be able to *hear* around corners, providing us with enough information to feel at ease and unthreatened. The greater the hearing impairment, the greater the disorientation. At night, if a child cries out, will the cry be heard? If a knock at the door brings a warning, will it be heard? Oftentimes—no. To this person, the wind only blows when standing in it. Rain only falls if it can be seen or felt. Crickets on a summer night do not exist at all.

We all need orientation. It is essential if we are to maintain that balance we have with our environment. We need input from auditory and visual stimuli to feel alive. We need to hear. We need to see. We need to feel human.

I am just as deaf as I am blind. The problems of deafness are deeper and more complex, if not more important than those of blindness. Deafness is a much worse misfortune. For it means the loss of the most vital stimulus—the sound of the voice that brings language, sets thoughts astir, and keeps us in the intellectual company of man.[6]

—HELEN KELLER

Chapter II
THE MEANING OF HEARING

I KNOW YOU BELIEVE YOU UNDERSTOOD WHAT YOU THOUGHT I SAID BUT WHAT YOU HEARD IS NOT WHAT I MEANT. This maxim is old. Words convey meaning and "meaning" is the result of a generally agreed upon arbitrary set of symbols. With the proper use of these symbols we have language. And with language we are able to express ourselves. It is a way of turning our thoughts inside out—it is external.

But language may also be internal. We all know that any child who develops normally will soon learn the meaning of the word "mommy," even before being able to utter the word. An infant develops inner language within the first year of life. He realizes that words are symbols of experiences before he can actually use any of the symbols (words) himself.

When a child can integrate the words he hears (such as you repeating "mommy"), and can understand them by what they represent in his own inner language, he has then developed receptive language. The child learns that he must take what he hears in the world out there, process it through his inner language, and finally try to say it so that he can belong to that communicative world that he knows exists. When our little child becomes capable of saying the words that he knows represent symbols in our world, he has achieved expressive language. Expressive language usually occurs in the second year of life and will necessarily lead to speech development at the same time.

The normal hearing child develops language as a result of auditory stimuli. But deaf and hard of hearing infants depend much more on visual and tactual stimuli to acquire language. For a child, a hearing loss may mean impaired speech and language development, as well as a host of other complications (emotional, mental, psychological, sociological, etc.). In the adult, even after the normal development of language, words must still be heard and understood if ideas are to be accurately expressed.

> . . . Words play an enormous part in our lives . . . . The old idea that words possess magical powers is false; but its falsity is the distortion of a very important truth. Words do have a magical effect—but not in the way that the magicians supposed, and not on the objects they were trying to influence. Words are magical in the way they affect the minds of those who use them. "A mere matter of words," we say contemptuously, forgetting that words have power to mould men's thinking, to canalize their feeling, to direct their willing and acting. Conduct and character are largely determined by the nature of the words we currently use to discuss ourselves and the world around us.[7]

—ALDOUS HUXLEY

NORMAL AND ABNORMAL HEARING

Normal hearing is defined in terms of a range of sound detection at various frequencies. Decibels are used to describe, measure and represent limits of deviation from normal. It is entirely possible to have a less sensitive hearing threshold than average and still be within the normal *range* of hearing.

Hence, hearing within the normal range can be defined as a status of audition whereby sound is received at the ear, is channeled through the auditory pathway without interference to the brain, and is interpreted and identified as the original message.

Once sound can no longer be properly channeled through the auditory system and is perceived incorrectly or not at all, reception of sound has become impaired. Hearing is then considered to be deficient. People who are unable to receive any meaningful auditory input are deaf. However, more than 33 million Americans suffer from a loss of meaningful sounds as a result of the ear's inability to transmit a complete message. If only part of a message is received, the condition is referred to as "hard of hearing." This is quite apart from being deaf.

THE AUDIOGRAM

An audiogram is a graphic representation of an individual's hearing threshold. It provides the otologist with diagnostic information and the audiologist with aural rehabilitative information. Threshold as plotted on an audiogram is that point at which sound is just barely audible 50 percent of the time. Threshold is represented with an X in Figures 1 and 2. In other words, the X represents where the sound of a tone is barely heard. Frequency (in cycles per second or more appropriately and recently referred to as Hertz, abbreviated Hz) and intensity (in decibels, abbreviated dB) are plotted on the audiogram. An

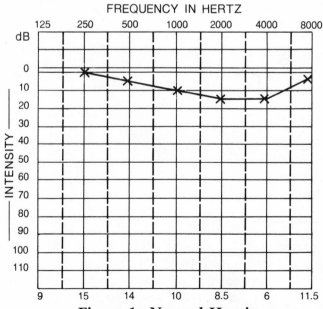

Figure 1. Normal Hearing

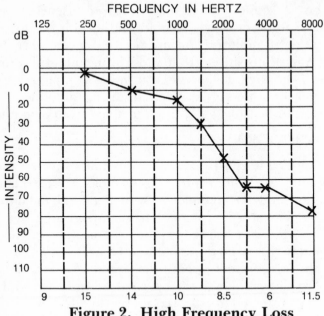

Figure 2. High Frequency Loss

audiogram measures the intensity (dB) and frequency (Hz) of hearing. The poorer the hearing, the greater the intensity needed to hear. "Normal" hearing is considered in terms of a range between −15 and +15 dB (or 0 dB). A mild hearing loss is 15 to 35 dB; moderate loss, 35 to 60 dB; severe loss, 60 to 85 dB; and a profound loss is considered greater than 85 dB.

Figure 1 represents hearing within normal limits at all frequencies tested. Figure 2 represents a typical high frequency sensorineural hearing loss found in the overwhelming majority of millions who suffer from hearing impairment caused by long-term noise exposure or the aging process (presbycusis).

SEE YOUR DOCTOR

If you have a hearing problem, the initial step is to see an ear specialist. He is a preferred physician over a general practitioner because of his particular training. An otologist (ear specialist), otolaryngologist (ear and throat specialist), and an otorhinolaryngologist (ear, nose and throat specialist) all are involved with medical care of the ear.

Often there is an audiologist working directly in practice with such physicians, available and qualified to evaluate hearing. A hearing test conducted in a room that has a high ambient noise level is unsatisfactory. It could provide the otologist with an inaccurate picture of hearing, which in turn could yield an incorrect diagnosis. A correct hearing examination is essential. Every patient should insist upon it (see Appendix I).

PERCENT OF HEARING LOSS

One of the first questions a patient will ask either an audiologist or a physician is: WHAT PERCENT OF HEARING LOSS DO I HAVE? The question has great merit, but the answer is sometimes very misleading.

A percent of hearing loss can be derived by an estimate of the number of damaged hair cells within the cochlea. There are approximately 12,000 hair cells, but calculating the percent of hearing loss in this way requires either removing the cochlea to examine the hair cells (hardly practical!), or photographing the microscopic hair cells by means of a photomicrograph—a costly method, and not as precise as an audiogram.

Hence, the audiogram has been used as the basis for determining percentage of hearing impairment. The amount of hearing loss in decibels is multiplied by a mathematical formula that reveals a percentage. THE AUDIOGRAM ITSELF DOES NOT REPRESENT A PERCENT OF HEARING LOSS. The method of representing hearing loss in terms of a percent was originally intended as a way of determining the amount of financial remuneration an individual with damaged hearing should receive. Generally, the greater the hearing loss, the greater the percentage and therefore the greater the amount of compensation.

Although percentage is still used to describe hearing loss for compensation, such a method is highly ambiguous when it comes to describing the actual problem of hearing. Percentage may work well for establishing guidelines of compensation, but it does not serve to clarify what has taken place in the ear and why there is often a problem of hearing without understanding.

When a figure of 30 percent is used, for example, it is not specified if the damage is in the lower, middle or upper frequencies for speech reception. WHERE the damage occurs determines the difficulty for speech intelligibility. This is the key factor in what you will hear. One thousand people may have a 30 percent loss of hearing and not one may have the same amount of loss within the same spectrum for speech. That is, one may have more damage in the lower frequencies, another more in the highs, and the various degrees in between are innumerable. One person may be far more impaired than the other, yet both may be informed that they have a 30 percent loss of hearing.

TRANSMISSION OF SOUND

The ear receives words and processes sound in a way that cannot be replicated by man. The transmission of sound is one of the most interesting and complex systems of all the senses. The changes that sound undergoes in the ear are like a journey into the universe, where still, in the midst of a booming technology, much is unknown.

The outer flap of the ear has always served to "capture" sound vibrations and channel them into the ear canal. However, prehistoric man probably benefited far more from this than modern man. Its primary purpose now seems to be to support hanging ornaments.

Sound makes five energy transformations in the ear. The acoustic vibrations (such as a person's voice) impinge upon the eardrum, setting the three tiny bones of the middle ear into motion. Once these bones (known as the malleus, incus, and stapes) are set into vibration, the first transformation of energy has taken place—from acoustic to mechanical energy. The second phase of energy conversion occurs at the oval window of the cochlea (a snail-shaped sensory end organ) that is filled with two fluids. The rocking motion of the three tiny bones pushes on the membrane covering the window into the cochlea, creating waves in the fluid-filled chambers. Once the fluid is set into motion, energy has changed from mechanical to hydraulic—the third transformation. Deep within the cochlea

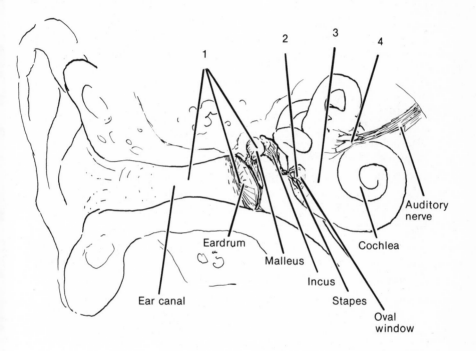

Figure 3: Stages in the transmission of sound.

1. Sound transformed into mechanical energy.
2. Mechanical energy creates waves at oval window.
3. Mechanical energy transformed into hydraulic energy.
4. Hydraulic energy is converted into electrical energy and transported along auditory nerve to brain.
5. (not shown) Electrical energy is interpreted as sound by brain.

rows of microscopic hair cells begin a shearing action as a result of the fluid motion. Once these hair cells begin to move, hydraulic energy is converted into electrical energy. The nervous system then picks up the message and takes it through the most complex and least understood transformation—neural energy—and onto the brain. Once sound has reached the brain via neurological pathways, the fifth and final conversion occurs, with psychological energy providing interpretation of the original signal.

TUNING IN

Tuning in is important (see chapter seven, question-answer number six). The ear must tune in sound like a radio receiver. The more frequencies received within the speech spectrum, and the stronger the signal, the greater the intelligibility of the message. If there is a breakdown at any of the five major auditory energy transforming centers, aural communication may become severely impaired.

The vast majority of people who have hearing problems suffer from a breakdown in the cochlea (the fourth energy-conversion station), where delicate hair cells have become injured. The sound of a single firecracker or shotgun may cause immediate and permanent damage. Hair cells of the inner ear are in groups. Therefore many hair cells may be affected by high intensities rather than a single hair cell reacting alone. If hair cells are damaged they will not respond to the motion of fluids that surround them, resulting in an incapacity to produce an electrical charge. If only a few hair cells are damaged, it may go undetected for a day, a year, or perhaps never noticed. But when enough hair cells are damaged, research has indicated that hearing will be impaired— permanently.

COMMUNICATION

Communication is the art of exchanging thoughts—a way of expressing or receiving ideas. A glance. A touch. A motion. A sigh. A word. Many words. No words. Man's communication system is based on verbal and non-verbal language and it has been believed for thousands of years that such a system is unique to man. But it is not. Dolphin research has shown that they have a highly sophisticated language—a language human beings as yet cannot decipher. Chimpanzees have been taught to communicate (non-verbally) with man and with other chimpanzees through symbol systems available through sign language and computers. Such breakthroughs in the recent past crumble the notion that language is unique to man. Only a few years ago, the idea of communicating with monkeys through a language system seemed absurd. Today communicating with extraterrestrial beings seems absurd. The future is certain to bring about great developments in communication.

MISSING COMPONENTS

The verbal human communication system functions on a high level of redundancy. That is, there is much more information within the message being conveyed than is actually necessary. "How are you?" is a typical greeting. However, often it is spoken "How-you?" without any loss of information. The mind fills in missing sounds that the ear does not (or cannot) pick up. Such auditory closure is unconscious. Visual closure is a counterpart that can be easily illustrated in the following example.

EXAMPLE I

Vou can read this without much difficulty

This message is easy to read because enough information is present even though the message itself is incomplete. Relative to the hearing impaired individual, if enough information is provided, the message may be received correctly. But when the primary message is altered greatly, it may not be comprehensible:

EXAMPLE II

Not all messages are unintelligible

Example II illustrates how the message may be obliterated when too much information is destroyed. The hearing impaired person may hear sounds easily, but the sound may be unintelligible. Just as with the visual counterpart in Example II, some information is available, but not enough to provide easy interpretation of the message itself. (Example II was: "Not all messages are unintelligible.")

How a message is presented may also affect the intelligibility of information being conveyed:

EXAMPLE III

$T^hu^rs{}^day$ $m{}_0{}^.{}_1{}^.{}_1{}_g$ $s_h{}^0u^ld$ $p_r{}_0{}_ve$ t^o b^e v^er^y $i^nt_er_e{}_st^in_g$. Here, the message is complete but the pattern has changed. This does not reduce the intelligibility of the information, but it may reduce the speed in which it can be perceived. If this pattern were used over and over again, it might become quite easy to read. Familiarity with the pattern is then very important. In a similar way, a person may speak with a heavy accent without impairing the message. Only the pattern of the information presented changes. If one is familiar with the pattern, the information is still available. It may simply require more time for the total information to be processed.

Speech sounds may be altered, distorted or omitted entirely without necessarily a loss of information, as illustrated. If you happen to be in a room with a live rock and roll band and see a friend approaching you, you may ask, "How are you?" Your friend might not have heard you because of the loud music, but chances are it was quite a predictable greeting and the response might be just as predictable. If your friend responds with an answer that is inaudible to you, you still may be able to receive the message through visual observation. Your friend may bite his lower lip, with the upper teeth protruding and the upper lip retracted, followed by a lowering of the jaw with an open mouth. You may never be consciously aware of these movements, but it's likely that you would know that your friend said "Fine."

Such visual observation of speech is little more than speechreading. It is the processing of information that occurs even in the most normal hearing individuals. Lip movements, tongue positions, facial expression and body language (movements or gestures) provide needed information, particularly in environments that have extremely high ambient noise levels when audition alone cannot account for reception of the total message. Since words can't be tasted or smelled, auditory and visual senses are the most important channels for effective communication.

VOWELS AND CONSONANTS

The human communication system in normal hearing people depends primarily upon audition—"The sound of the voice that brings language. . . ."[8] These sounds comprise vowels and consonants. The human ear receives vowels at frequencies *below* 1000 Hz, while consonants are primarily *above* 1000 Hz. Therefore, you can see how impairment of hearing at various frequencies may impair certain sounds. Research investigations have revealed that when sounds below 400 Hz remain intact with sounds above 400 Hz eliminated, the message is nearly impossible to decipher. In such a low frequency loss, the majority of vowel energy is inaudible making speech unintelligible. When frequencies above 1000 Hz are eliminated, many consonants are severely affected, producing a significant reduction in the discrimination of the message.

The sound /e/ when spoken (as in sp*ee*d) vibrates the throat. Say it. Feel your throat vibrate. It is a vowel sound with energy in the lower frequencies. The vocal cords are responsible for the production of vowel sounds. The cords vibrate at a speed that exceeds the near-invisible flutter of a hummingbird's wings.

The sound of /sh/ (as in *sh*e) consists of two consonants and occurs in the higher frequencies within the speech spectrum. Say it. It sounds like you are telling someone to "hush"—"SH!" Feel your throat. It may not even move. There is no vocal cord activity and the sound may be extremely difficult to detect with a high frequency hearing loss. It may sound very similar to /f/, /th/, /t/, or /s/. Say the sounds. They are audibly quite similar and may be confused even by the normal hearing person. Therefore, a word such as "she" may be misunderstood by a person with a hearing loss in the high frequencies. It may easily sound like "he" or "e," since the /sh/ could be difficult to hear.

27

Hence, we realize that vowels are low frequency sounds and consonants are high frequency sounds.

HIGH FREQUENCY HEARING LOSS

The number one hearing problem around the world is a high frequency sensorineural one. The cause is exposure to noise (as well as presbycusis, a loss that occurs with age).

As explained in the previous section, consonants occur in the higher frequencies and therefore a loss in this range will impair the reception of these sounds. Also as demonstrated earlier in this chapter, some parts of a message can be totally eliminated without impairing the message itself. But when too much information is lost, the message will be difficult to interpret.

The speech organs are capable of producing more than 700 different sounds. The English language utilizes less than 50 sounds to allow us to utter all of the hundreds of thousands of words in our language. Learning some languages will be more difficult than others because some utilize more high frequency sounds than others. Hence, if you have a high frequency hearing loss, it would be more difficult for you to learn (and hear the sounds of) French than Japanese.

A rather small percentage of all the people afflicted with hearing impairment have strictly a low frequency loss. In such cases, voices will tend to sound like loud whispers, with a lot of crispness in the sound, but not much intensity, since the vowels contain all the primary energy and thus carrying power. Intelligible speech is not possible through either vowels or consonants alone. It is the interaction of both that provide speech to the normal ear.

POOR HAROLD

"For God's sake, Harold! Why don't you listen more carefully?"

"All right, I'm sorry. I didn't hear you. You wanna try it again?"

"I add, Harold, that firty year we been sane and you've all gone to top oh ought ten a hook a young grrrrr! Phew! I'b add it, air old!"

Poor Harold. He has a high frequency hearing loss, making consonant sounds indistinguishable and misinterpreted. Although he may be guilty of his wife's accusation, he can't get to first base with a defense if he can't make out what it is she "mumbled." The heaviest complaint wailed by hard of hearing persons is that "people mumble." Indeed, perhaps somewhat surprisingly, most people speak rather clearly, or at least distinctly enough to be understood. But those with hearing problems (particularly with a high frequency impairment) report that others sound like they need lessons on how to speak—but there may be lessons in store on how to hear.

Harold's wife was complaining about his behavior. She was a little upset and was not speaking directly to him. Besides that, the dishwasher was on and he was at the opposite end of the kitchen. She stated: "I said, Harold, that thirteen years we've been sailing and you have the gall to stop so often and look at the young girls! Well! I've had it, Harold!"

And Harold has had it too. He can't hear well anymore. But then, Harold thinks to himself, "Why bother to hear this?" But there's more, much more that he is missing. Harold serves as an example of what can happen with high frequency hearing loss. Speech can sound so chopped up, so obliterated, that regardless of repetitions, the level of frustration remains high because the facility to receive sound in the ear has been partially destroyed. Rather than a *repeat,* Harold needs information *re-phrased.* Repeating the same words only presents the identical problem again. In Harold, as in millions, the condition of his hearing loss is permanent.

Chapter III
NOISE:
THE INVISIBLE POLLUTION

You rise in the morning, startled into reality by the obscene ring of an alarm clock. The first room you head for is the bathroom. where implements of destruction await you: an electric shaver, an electric comb or brush, an electric toothbrush, a vibrator, a cap gun (that comes with a noisy child). The sink may jerk arrhythmically due to faulty plumbing and the faucet may produce an indescribable squeal from vibrations when the water runs.

You know the family's in the kitchen. You can hear the dog howling in harmony with the garbage disposal as last night's munchies are destroyed. You flush the toilet which takes five minutes to stop hissing and then you head for the kitchen. You know it's time to eat because the dishwasher has already gone into rinse cycle. An all-new, all-purpose, all-electric blender is beating eggs in the kitchen to the quadraphonic sound of the Berlin Philharmonic Orchestra in the living room. A radio is blaring the morning news from a bedroom and the children are shouting at each other in the den as they watch T.V. in anticipation of another smog alert. The cacophony of the morning is enough to drive you back beneath the sheets, except that a cat, a turtle and your four-year-old have taken over the bedroom. The baby in the high chair is banging her tin cup on the table in hope of more milk. Fred is driving up in his truck. You know it's Fred because of the mufflers. You no sooner put a fork to the eggs, the end result of half the kitchen noise, when

Fred starts blasting the horn and it's not even eight o'clock yet. Reflexively you grab a coat, put your ulcer back in your stomach and race for the door. Your wife (whose head is buried deeply beneath a portable high-speed electric hair curler) hands you your keys and extends a warm kiss. But she vibrates your teeth from the hair curler that encompasses her head and just before your gums bleed she downshifts her futuristic twelve-speed machine to wave you good morning!

Indeed, every household may not be so dramatic, rushed or neurotic, but certainly the "average" household suffers from the dilemma of noise above tolerable levels. With the advent of chain saws and power mowers, the unmuffled minibike, snowmobiles and the like, the future is not bright in a world where noise increases year by year. This is reflected in the loss of hearing among millions of Americans. It is just one sensory reaction to man's procreated environment.

NOISE DEFINED

Noise is classically defined as "unwanted sound" but may more appropriately be defined as "potentially damaging unwanted sound." Such unwanted sound did not begin with the first clap of thunder nor with prehistoric man shouting obscenities from treetops. For all intents and purposes, noise began with the Industrial Revolution in the 1700's. It has been increasing steadily on an upward continuum ever since. Certainly undesirable noises can be traced as far back in time as B.C., when Ezekiel spoke of "noise of tumult" or when Amos complained that musicians were playing too loudly (Bible translations).

WHO SUFFERS?

Early in the 1960's, the United States Public Health Service announced that the problem of hearing was then the nation's most chronic handicapping disability. It still is 15 years later. Hearing loss can be so slow that it can actually happen without great awareness as in the cases of partial hearing loss confined to the higher frequencies. There are more people afflicted with hearing problems that are permanent than all the people in the

United States afflicted with blindness, multiple sclerosis, tuberculosis, kidney disease, liver disease, venereal disease and cancer COMBINED!

In a world so full of sound, we can no longer be deceived that high intensities are harmless. On the contrary, literature in the fields of hearing, acoustics, psychoacoustics and medicine is replete with information based on scores of research studies and data that reveal the true harmful effects of noise.

THE DECIBEL

It is not intended that you be boggled with mathematical formulas or technicalities for a reasonable understanding of what "intensity" is. Noise (sound) is measured in decibels (dB). For a better understanding of the decibel as used in measurement of sound intensity: rustling of leaves is about 20 dB; a soft whisper at five feet approximately 25 dB; average conversational speech is 60 dB; a jackhammer, 90 to 110 dB; live rock and roll music, 90 to 130 dB; a U.S. Army tactical launcher at 400 feet, 134 dB; the roar of a jet aircraft as it speeds into the air upon take-off, approximately 140+ dB at several hundred feet; a U.S. Army Sargent Missile at 100 feet, 145 dB; a bazooka fired at one foot, 163 dB; a 105 mm. Howitzer, 190 dB.

EAR PROTECTION

Standard earplugs of rubber are not adequate in many situations, and cotton is never recommended since it is ineffective. Most soft silicone earplugs will attenuate sound approximately 15 to 35 dB, depending upon the frequency of the stimulus. An earplug of cottonwool soaked in paraffin may reduce noise by 20 to 30 dB. Earmuffs (ear defenders) can often reduce noise levels by 40 to 45 dB. There is an earplug available made of a soft foamlike material that can be rolled into a ball and placed in the ear, expanding once in the ear. This can reduce noise up to 50 dB at some frequencies.

A noise level of 120 dB produces great discomfort for most human beings. Exposure to a Howitzer (190 dB) may easily rupture both eardrums and produce instantaneous permanent hearing loss upon the very first shot. Protection against such devastating noise emissions is not possible. There simply is no means of protection available. Maximum ear protection reduces the level of sound hitting the ear by only 50 dB at best. Therefore, in the example of Howitzer noise emissions, even with ear protection, sound levels of 140+ dB still reach the ear and can still produce immediate and permanent damage.

For people exposed to levels around 120 dB (area of discomfort), effective ear defenders or earplugs* can decrease such harmful levels at certain frequencies. However, not all frequencies are protected. In excess of 120 dB of noise the skull carries dangerous noise levels by bone conduction through the head and into the ear, so that even the best available protection is not sufficient.

The major drawback to ear protection of any kind is that it may prevent hearing warning signals, and it can prevent workers from communicating with each other. Lack of communication has been shown to produce feelings of frustration, anger, strain and other emotional problems. For many people earplugs or ear defenders produce headaches and/or dizziness, even after short-term use, as a result of sensory deprivation. Thus, ear protection from noise exposure presents a serious dilemma.

Russia has recognized "acoustic trauma" (noise-induced hearing loss from an impulsive sound) as an occupational disease since 1929. Many other countries are aware of such impairment and consider it more serious than the United States does. English law still does not recognize this problem. Boilermakers in England continue working without compensation for their severe impairment to hearing.

PHONY EAR PROTECTOR

One of the non-medical myths concerning the ear is a recent "scientifically developed" ear protection device. This device claims to have a sophisticated miniature high frequency filter allowing an individual to be exposed to loud noises without damaging the higher frequencies of the ear. It also

*Ear defenders or earplugs are available through most hearing aid offices.

claims that normal conversation can be conducted with the unit in place in the ear canal. This is unsubstantiated and is as much misleading as it is fraudulent. I ran an experiment in 1974 and repeated it in 1975 using this product. Twenty normal hearing individuals were given a hearing test. Threshold was established. Hearing was found to be normal at all the frequencies tested. The unit was placed in the test ears and the subjects remained in the soundproof room and were tested.

Results indicated that the unit caused a decrease at all frequencies tested. *However,* the product proved to decrease hearing more in the lower frequencies than in the higher frequencies. For the sake of humor, a piece of chewing gum was wrapped in tissue and used to plug the test ear of the original subjects (the gum was already chewed). The gum proved to be more effective than the filtering unit at all but one of the frequencies tested. The device can actually be quite dangerous since people purchase the unit believing the advertisements that claim protection against gunfire or sudden loud sounds. It is not as effective as it purports to be. Hearing loss certainly can still result with its use in high noise areas. Beware! The product is still being marketed.

MAXIMUM TOLERABLE NOISE

It is difficult to determine exactly how much abuse the human ear can withstand before malfunctioning. Noise in excess may well act to weaken the ear, making it more susceptible to future insult. At the same time, such an ear may check out as "normal" although it may be badly weakened. The Occupational Safety and Health Administration (OSHA) has provided what they consider to be *safe limits* of noise exposure with maximum allowable time of exposure and actual levels: eight hours at 90 dB; six hours at 92 dB; four hours at 95 dB; two hours at 100 dB; one hour at 105 dB; thirty minutes at 110 dB; fifteen minutes or less at 115 dB; 120 dB considered loud enough to produce a hearing loss.[9] If the time of exposure to any of these intensities is exceeded, the risk of hearing damage is immediately increased.[10,11] This method of determining safe limits of exposure to loud intensities is questionable, because the delicate microscopic hair follicles of the inner ear can become more easily fatigued as noise exposure at these levels and time periods continues on a daily basis. Hence, the more fatigued ear may be more likely to result in impairment than a non-fatigued ear.[12] However, there is a great lack of research on this point.

HEADPHONES AND EARPIECES

Earmolds shaped to fit a particular ear are widely used by telephone operators, news media including both radio and television, engineers, musicians and producers in recording and movie studios, police departments, etc. These individually designed earmolds or even simple headsets carry sound directly to the eardrum. Listening to any stimulus through one of these units has reduced the distance that sound travels from perhaps several feet to two inches. When sound travels directly from an earpiece, it impinges upon the eardrum and cannot be absorbed in anything else. Sound waves from a speaker are absorbed or refracted in everything in its path (such as drapes, carpeting, sofas, chairs, lamps, tables and even people). Therefore, when listening to sound from a speaker, the stimulus does not impinge directly upon the eardrum. An 85 dB sound source coming through an earpiece is far more hazardous than 85 dB of sound coming from a speaker in a well furnished room. However, the trend of using such earpieces is just beginning. It may take years before their damage is fully realized.

WHO'S IN DANGER?

Traditionally, weavers, braziers, boilermakers, railroad workers and blacksmiths have been infamous for their trades that have caused total deafness. Noise is on the increase. Growth in industry is also on the increase (barring times of recession). It can be expected that the problem will get much worse before the trend reverses itself. Specialists in many fields have reported that damage to hearing usually begins to taper off after 10 to 15 years of exposure. The greatest amount of damage is therefore incurred within the first 10 years, and more so, the first few years when noise may begin to weaken the ears' ability to resist additional abuses. One is more likely to suffer loss after the age of 30.

The three most important factors relevant to noise are: 1) the intensity, 2) the length of time exposed and 3) the frequencies at which the noise occurs. It must be stressed that noise as a cause of hearing loss is not restricted to industrial workers. A lawn mower thrusts out a hardy 110+ dB. Exposure to this for longer than 30 minutes (according to OSHA standards) is dangerous. Perhaps such products should come with an engraving, "The Surgeon General has determined that mowing lawns may be hazardous to your health."

MUSIC AS DANGEROUS SOUND

The average estimate of today's rock and roll music in any given discotheque is approximately 110 dB at a distance of one to twenty feet from the speakers.[13] Based on OSHA standards, excess of thirty minutes exposure to such cacophony should be considered hazardous to hearing. Research has indicated that there is first a temporary threshold shift (TTS) in hearing. The temporary loss in hearing may last from a few hours to a few weeks and upon further exposure may become a permanent threshold shift (PTS), making it impossible for the ear to completely recuperate from such abuse. People regularly listen to live rock music at levels exceeding 110 dB for several hours (well beyond OSHA's thirty-minute limit).[14]

One of many research projects studied the effects of high intensity music on chinchillas. After exposure to 123 dB of music, some animals showed a PTS of 50 dB or more.[15] If humans had this amount of loss at the frequencies necessary for the reception of speech, a hearing aid would be needed to properly understand ordinary conversational speech.

Photomicrography is a process of photographing the microscopic structures of the body. The fine hair cells of the inner ear have been studied through investigations on lower animals and man using this method. Live rock and roll music was recorded on tape in one study and found to be 122 dB. A tape loop was made providing continuous music to guinea pigs.

Protective earplugs were used until the 65th hour of exposure at which point the right plug was removed and the tape played for another 33 hours. At the completion of the experiment, the inner ears of the animals were removed and inspected. A photomicrograph of the left (protected) ear showed normal unaltered structures. The right ear (exposed 33 hours) showed scarring and collapsed walls of the inner ear with 10 percent damage to inner rows of hair cells. The outer hair cells for hearing were 20 percent damaged. Hence, more than one-quarter of the total cell population was severely damaged in the exposed ears.[16]

CHILDREN WITH HEARING PROBLEMS

In the mid 1960's, a study on 1,000 school age children in Colorado revealed more boys with high frequency hearing impairments than girls.[17] As many as 11 percent of the ninth graders suffered permanent losses. Approximately three million young school-age children suffer from serious hearing disorders that, if left untreated, could become permanent.[18] This amounts to 10 percent of all the children enrolled in public schools in the United States. It was assumed that more boys than girls revealed hearing losses in the Colorado study from their exposure to generally louder music as well as exposure to guns and rifles, firecrackers, carpentry and head blows from body contact sports. Such losses can be directly attributable to home and recreational environments.

DENTISTS

Research has revealed that large areas of hair cells in the cochlea (hearing mechanism) are destroyed by many sources that might otherwise seem harmless. Dentists have proposed that high-level music has an anesthetic quality putting patients into a light hypnotic state. Some have even used it through headphones as a tranquilizing element instead of using topical anesthesia. However, due to the evidence of noise-induced hearing loss from music, it was eliminated. An unpublished study of mine in New York in 1971 revealed that dentists in the group that I investigated suffered from hearing impairments at the corresponding frequencies to their dental drills (in this case, 2000 Hz).

INDUSTRIAL WORKERS

The U.S. Department of Labor estimates that approximately 75 million Americans were employed in industry in 1971. Of that group, about 25 percent were exposed to levels intense enough to cause permanent hearing loss (90+ dB). This is substantiated by further research (and shows the figure of 25 percent to be conservative). Research reveals that *at least* 25 percent of those who apply for industrial jobs have a *significant* hearing loss (with some studies reporting incidences of 50 percent and higher). With this in mind, and using the statistic of 25 percent, no fewer than 18 million Americans in industry alone have hearing losses.[19]

GUNS AND THE DAMAGE DONE

Hunting is still a "Great American Sport." The National Rifle Association estimates that 20 million Americans are actively involved in hunting. The sound of gunshots can impair hearing as quickly as pulling the trigger.[20] The Eisenhower Commission on gun control in 1968 established that there are approximately 210 million firearms in circulation within the U.S. Handguns account for 45 million weapons with a rate of increase of approximately two and one-half million new purchases each year (or one new handgun bought every 13 seconds).

Hunters in general do not utilize ear defenders (earmuffs) and tend to buy commercially advertised earplugs that prove highly inadequate (see "Phony Ear Protector," p. 34). The level of sound from handguns reaches 160 dB.[21] OSHA reports that impulsive noise such as gunfire should never exceed 140 dB *at any time.*

One study in the 1960's reported that 500 soldiers assigned to a Mechanized Infantry Division were examined audiologically and all were found to be in very good health (including normal hearing). The average age was 36. All 500 men developed hearing losses in the higher frequencies following various periods of intense noise exposure. Additional complaints consisted of tinnitus (ringing in the ears) and pain when exposed to loud noises in the future (recruitment). The levels to which they were exposed ranged as high as 190 dB, as in the sound emitted from a Howitzer.[22]

In 1971, the Surgeon General of the United States Army revealed the results of a Medical Research and Development Command.* Their investigation indicated that approximately 60 percent of all the men with 10+ years of active duty in the infantry, artillery and armor branches suffered from permanent hearing losses. Twenty-three to forty-one percent of the men were so impaired that they required mandatory duty limitations.

OUR ENVIRONMENT AND NOISE

A subway ride in New York City exceeds noise levels of 90 dB. A joy ride on the freeway in a convertible can reach 95 dB and higher, depending upon speed (and other factors). There are more than 180 million road travelers in the United States. Surveys have shown that transportation-related sources are responsible for the highest level of community noises. The intensity of sound generally increases with the speed and weight of a vehicle. The average automobile that doubles its speed (e.g., from 30 to 60 mph) will nearly triple the level of acoustic energy produced. Motorcycles quadruple their intensity level when doubling their speed. The primary source of the noise pollution comes from the engine. Other major contributing factors include exhaust noises and tire-road noises. Surveys have shown that the quietest hours are between midnight and five A.M. Environmental noises increase continually from five A.M. until eleven P.M. at which point a tapering off occurs. The greatest intensities occur at peak traffic hours at eight A.M. and five P.M. Depending on the weather, environmental noise levels may be lower in certain parts of the country. For example, snow acts to absorb sound. Also fewer people are

---

*Presented at the 86th Annual Meeting of the Acoustical Society of America, Los Angeles, California, October-November 1973.

likely to drive on snowy streets. This may account for lower daytime noise levels in January than in September in many parts of the country. The greatest contributors to nighttime noises are air conditioners and intermittent disturbances from emergency vehicles, street sweepers and barking dogs.[23,24]

AIR TRAFFIC

The convenience of flying has become an integral part of the American way of life. The noise emissions from aircraft are accepted frequently as a necessary evil. In suburbia-America, you may occasionally see an aircraft flying in the distance. You may smile to yourself and think of all the progress since the days of the horse and buggy. But imagine the sound of three million horses in the sky at one moment in time—indeed, a Pegasus's nightmare.

Plans are continuing for the development and production of the Super Sonic Transport (SST), the fastest of the superplanes, capable of more noise emission than any other commercial aircraft. The two and one-half billion dollar machine flies literally as fast as a bullet. Clipping along 12 miles high and greater than twice the speed necessary to break the sound barrier, the sonic boom is merely one by-product of this technological freak. It can produce multiple shock waves audible in excess of 60 miles.

In the meantime, Boeing Corporation is hiring deaf individuals (requiring complete deafness in order to be hired) to work around extremely high noise levels, such as welding and riveting. The deaf communicate easily with one another by the use of sign language. They therefore would not be subjected to the danger of hearing loss nor the frustration of not being able to communicate with one another on the job where noise levels are high. However, they are still subjected to nearly all of the physiological effects produced by noise (to be discussed later in this chapter).[25]

The 1975 Aircraft Award (which I give with humor since awards are a sign of the times) goes to Chicago's O'Hare International Airport for breaking the world's record of greatest number of landings and take-offs in one place

(668,368). O'Hare has been the busiest airport in the world for nearly 20 years (excluding military air bases). In recent years, there have been no New York airports that have even ranked in the top ten busiest. But in California, six of the top ten busiest airports in the world are within a 30-mile radius of Los Angeles alone.

Air traffic is similar to street traffic in that there are peak periods, but if an average were taken, there would be at least one flight every 12 seconds around Los Angeles, or more than 300 flights every hour, 24 hours around the clock, every day of every month all year round. Los Angeles International Airport was the sixth busiest airport in the world in 1975 with 455,836 landings and take-offs. Somewhat frightening is the fact that air traffic is increasing at a rate of six to seven percent each year (excluding years of national economic decline). Farmers in the backlands of Montana may not be very interested in legislation for noise abatement but millions of citizens in cities around the United States (and the world) are exposed to as many as hundreds of daily flights low over their homes, causing property damage as well as extremely high ambient noise levels.

Aircraft noise from the Los Angeles International Airport is audible in excess of 10 miles from the airport and has increased environmental noise more than 10-fold.

A major breakthrough occurred in February 1975, when the City Court of Los Angeles allocated in excess of one million dollars to 552 families in the airport vicinity for noise fall-out from airport traffic. Several more major cases have followed suit.

There are four major flight paths directly over Los Angeles that alone affect at least three million citizens. There is even a flight path over one of the wealthiest areas in Los Angeles—Beverly Hills. Planes routinely fly below 5,000 feet on this path. It is not uncommon for these people to experience incredible intensities within their homes as a result of air traffic even with all windows and doors closed! YOUR CITY IS NO DIFFERENT!

There are noise ordinances in effect in nearly all parts of

the United States. All of the ordinances describe exactly how much "too much" noise is and then it is left up to the jury or judge to determine actual violations. California has one of the most stringent municipal codes in the United States. One of these more rigid codes just happens to affect a residential area directly under a flight path near the Los Angeles International Airport. Residents are prohibited by law to produce noise levels in excess of 60 dB during the day and 50 dB at night. Any violation is considered a misdemeanor with a maximum fine of not more than five hundred dollars and/or a jail sentence of not more than six months. Aircraft exceed the limits set by this ordinance both during the day and at night. Yet homeowners are expected (and forced) to comply with such regulations. The Federal Aviation Administration (FAA) is fully aware of the violations incurred daily in and around the Los Angeles International Airport, but neither they nor those enforcing the laws have taken any action to resolve the noise problem. One estimate reports that more than 1,000 aircraft break the residential ordinances daily. If such an ordinance were in effect under all four flight paths and assuming prosecution were undertaken, more than one billion dollars would be rung up in fines alone in one year not to mention imprisonment of FAA executives for such violations.[26]

LOW-LEVEL DISTURBING SOUNDS

Not everybody is affected by noise. Some people appear to have greater or lesser tolerances for noise. Millions of people confronted with noise pollution also face the psychological, physiological and sociological anomalies associated with high intensities. Noise is considered to be a stressor. The military ranks noise as the primary source of stress to servicemen. The aversive reactions to disturbing sounds even at relatively low intensities can be observed by its annoying effects: the screech of chalk across a blackboard; squealing tires; broken glass; the sound of soft music, but music you dislike; continual ringing of a doorbell or telephone; a cough in a movie theater; somebody in a library bouncing a just-sharpened pencil tip on a wooden table; the sound of a mosquito near the ear in the middle of the night. All of these sounds are disturbing to many people, but are not at high intensity levels. With the added factor of intensity, the psychological reaction is far more dramatic.

PSYCHOLOGICAL EFFECTS OF NOISE

The psychological effects of noise on man are extremely difficult to evaluate because the effects are so subtle. In September 1975, a total of $86,800 was paid for mental and emotional damages to 41 individuals living in the Greater Westchester area north of the Los Angeles International Airport. The emotional and mental conditions described by the victims included annoyance, irritability, nervousness, fear, frustration, anger, worry and strain. Research supports these claims, revealing that noise can produce feelings of uneasiness, discomfort, tension, anxiety, aggression and fatigue.[27-34] It was also reported that the noise from low-flying commercial aircraft (landing and taking off) produced hearing loss and prevented or restricted daily activities within the home (such as children doing homework, telephone conversations, enjoying radio and television programs, sleeping, and enjoying sexual relations).

The damaging psychological effects of noise may extend much further into our lives than we are ready to admit. Noise has motivated murderers in various cities in the United States, according to newspaper reports. Man is unquestionably the most adaptive of all animals, capable of suppressing tremendous emotional responses. But inhibition of otherwise expressive-behavioral reactions can cause both psychological and physiological problems. The man working on a job he dislikes suppresses his discontentment and develops an ulcer. Another man working on a job where noise is so loud that he cannot communicate with fellow workers suffers from frustration, anxiety (and other symptomatic reactions already discussed) and takes them home with him at the end of the day—to his wife and children! A study on steel mill workers revealed that they had great difficulty with relationships in their lives at work and at home as a result of the high intensity of noise in their working environments. Another study showed that 50 percent of the subjects displayed obvious neuroses and emotional disturbances related to their exposure to noise at work.

PHYSIOLOGICAL EFFECTS OF NOISE

The physiological reactions to noise have been proved on animals including man. Noise can cause vasoconstriction (a narrowing of the blood vessels) in man, allowing less blood to flow to certain parts of the body (including the ear) that depend on a regular flow for nourishment. If the cochlea does not receive sufficient blood supply, cell degeneration is inevitable, resulting in hearing loss.

Increased flow of adrenalin is a direct result of noise insult.[35] This has been correlated with migraine headaches[36] and fatigue.[37] Research studies have shown incredible physiological reactions to noise in rats,[38] mice,[39] guinea pigs,[40] rabbits,[41] dogs, honeybees,[42] farm animals (sheep, horses, cattle)[43] and wildlife.[44] The effects have included increased pulse rate[45] and adreno-cortical activity;[46] stomach constriction;[47] changes in the hypothalamus,[48] respiration,[49] heart rate,[50] blood pressure[51] and fertilization;[52] gastric ulcers;[53] lung hemorrhages; effects on the lipid and cholesterol metabolism;[54] and a decrease in thymus glands[55] and changes in brain chemistry.[56]

A group of rats exposed to noise in one study showed far greater difficulty with maze learning than the control group.[57] However, the group in this study that had the difficulty was exposed to noise *in a prenatal state*—that is, before their birth. Therefore, this suggests the possible damaging effects which noise may have on a human fetus. Such a Pandora's box may well lead to discovering that noise can hinder psychological, physiological and neurological growth of a fetus. The human fetus is actually capable of hearing environmental sounds external to the womb by the twelfth week. A pregnant woman after her third month of pregnancy may be causing her unborn child a host of problems that she may not realize. Certainly, it could be suggested that a fetus exposed to loud rock and roll music may not develop as "normally" as if it had not been exposed to such high intensities. Since man develops so many

45

aversive reactions to loud sounds, it is only logical to assume that a fetus, a more susceptible and fragile being, would be just as ill-fated.

In another study, the mammary glands of rabbits became enlarged when exposed to loud noises. The enlargement resulted in the secretion of an abundance of milk, as though the rabbit had actually experienced a pregnancy when in fact it had not. The acoustic stimuli alone brought about physiological changes in the uterus and ovaries![58]

In still another study (and they go on and on), guinea pigs were exposed to paper caps fired from a toy gun.[59] Profound damage occurred to the microscopic hair cells of the inner ear at the corresponding frequencies to the caps. Another study showed that ultrasonic sound bombardment (above 18,000 Hz) to mice at high intensities raised their body temperatures so high that it killed them.[60]

The effects of noise pollution on wildlife are least understood because studying them in their natural habitat involves great difficulty. However, many creatures of nature depend upon the acuity of their hearing for homing, mating and predator detection. Man's interference has already proven to be detrimental.[61]

THE PRESS

The Washington Post, The Evening Star & News and *The Wall Street Journal* have reported on the problem of noise, yet their very own pressmen grinding out the printed news are exposed to levels of sound that are well in excess of safe limits. More than 50 percent of the pressmen from these three newspapers have suffered hearing impairments in at least one frequency related to their hazardous noisy work environments.[62]

THE EPA

The Environmental Protection Agency (EPA) established an office of Noise Abatement and Control in 1970 to protect humans from humans. The EPA is not a policing agency. Enforcement of regulations set forth by the EPA is expected to be handled at the individual state level.

For example, the EPA set forth regulations governing the noise emissions from interstate motor carriers (enacted on October 29, 1974). The EPA predicted that this would decrease the noise impact for approximately 10 million people. However, since enforcement of regulations by the EPA must occur at the city or state level, compliance is not guaranteed.

The inconsistencies within the governmental agencies themselves are even more disappointing. That is, on the one hand, we hear from OSHA that exposure to 90 dB for eight hours is the maximum limit. Yet the EPA has set forth the motor carrier regulation that *permits* 90 dB of noise emission at 50 feet or more and at 35 mph or more. But the drivers of these trucks are exposed to greater than 90 dB since they are much less than 50 feet from the noise (engines, tires, mufflers, air horns). Therefore, while this regulation may possibly lower environmental noise, it does not serve to adequately decrease the risk of injury to hearing (particularly to the drivers), which is the whole point of the regulation! It is important for such inconsistencies to be cleared up so that an effective program for noise control can begin.

COMPENSATION AND SALARY LOSS

There is a wide range of compensation for hearing loss in the United States—from thirty-three thousand dollars in the state of Arizona under workmen's compensation for total loss of hearing due to occupational conditions, to states such as Michigan and Ohio where no compensation is allocated for anything less than total loss in one ear. In the state of Pennsylvania, where industry provides more employment for miners than Arizona, workmen's compensation is not granted for total loss of hearing in one ear—the loss must be in both. The state of Ohio pays a maximum of fourteen hundred dollars for total loss of hearing in one ear while Arizona pays eleven thousand dollars (and Pennsylvania pays nothing). The disparity among states is great. Arizona certainly would seem a rather unlikely area for developing hearing loss while coal miners and steel workers in Pennsylvania are losing their hearing every year *without appropriate compensation*.[63] It is estimated that two million dollars per day is paid in workmen's compensation for noise-related injuries, lost man-hours and decreased efficiency.[64]

The first claims for hearing damage were levied against Bethlehem Steel in New York State during the 1940's. If workmen's compensation does not cover hearing impairment caused by occupational hazards, it would seem acceptable to initiate personal litigation against major industries who have been unwilling to claim responsibility for such damage. The success of litigation is quite high, but then it should be—the price of hearing loss is high. The Veterans Administration paid over forty-three million dollars in 1962 for compensation due to hearing loss alone.[65] The Department of Health, Education and Welfare estimates that the loss of earnings due to communicative disorders is more than one and one-half billion dollars annually.

CONSERVATION

Hearing conservation programs are a must in every aspect of industry. Earmuffs should be worn without hesitation and provided at no expense to every employee exposed to hazardous noise. This does not only include those working on the particular job, but anyone close enough to endanger their hearing. In one major aircraft production facility in the United States, secretaries, bookkeepers, and general office workers were exposed indirectly to high level jet engines since only a wall separated them from the noise. One woman spent over 20 years at the same job (with high noise levels beyond the protective wall) and developed a serious high frequency hearing loss for which workmen's compensation denied remuneration. This particular secretary began personal litigation with my support and received a "reasonable" financial settlement. How much money is "reasonable" for such a permanent sensory deprivation is rather debatable.

Employees should insist upon taking protection with the intent of saving their own hearing and not merely to appease an employer. Education about the effects of noise on hearing and other natural bodily functions is necessary. This should include informing women of damage resulting from exposure to high-speed blenders, garbage disposals, hair dryers, etc. Men working with power tools such as saws and drills are producing high frequency hearing losses. The affliction is not reversible. It doesn't go away like a cold. It stays. The EPA has not yet set forth regulations for such control and protection. Once they do, hopefully they will be able to help enforce noise abatement programs better than present controls in other governmental areas of noise.

All employees on any job should have a routine hearing evaluation by a clinical audiologist or person trained in the methods and techniques of hearing testing. Since noise-induced hearing loss usually strikes the higher frequencies first, these frequencies are of the utmost concern in industrial testing and should be checked routinely at intervals determined by the level of noise and the length of time exposed to the noise.

On July 8, 1974, *Time* magazine reported that industry would have to spend thirty-one billion dollars to lower factory noise in the U.S. by five dB. This amount of decrease is less than lowering the volume of an average stereo player or radio by one notch (or number). With such expenditures involved in the reduction of noise, industry is not yet in a great hurry to begin such conservation. But they may be forced into it eventually because hearing loss in industry is as inevitable as the present issues of air and water pollution.

POLLUTION

Man should have learned that pollution is a serious problem after the experience of radiation from nuclear bombs and leaks from nuclear reactors; from pesticides that kill humans as well as insects and frequently prove ineffective due to insect adaptation; from the air and water pollutants shed by automobiles and industry that cloud every major city in America; from the problem of solid wastes that are now regurgitating from the floors of oceans; and from dangerous gases created by the miles of massive landfills used as dumps. Noise has not yet been taken seriously perhaps because of its devious and sometimes inconspicuous way of developing. And too often it is not considered serious when, in fact, it is.

It has taken many years on the part of researchers to convince people that noise is a major problem—an element in the environment to be extremely aware of and take necessary protection from; an element that can be prevented if the proper steps are taken immediately.

WHAT IS NORMAL?

"Normal" is defined as the average, the common or the usual. If hearing loss occurs in enough people, it will become "normal." Any abnormality that people of a culture develop ceases to be classified as abnormal or subnormal at a point when the majority of people suffer from the affliction. The common cold is only "common" because it is normal for most people to experience it. Hearing loss is on the increase, has been, and is predicted to continue. The factors causing the losses are also going unchecked and getting louder year by year. If enough people eventually suffer from severe high frequency hearing impairment, it will not be thought of as unusual, uncommon or abnormal, but quite normal for the circumstances.

WHAT IS ABNORMAL?

The slow transition of making an abnormal physical state "normal" is happening NOW! The civil service has been changing their requirements as often as every six months to allow more and more candidates with high frequency hearing impairments to be considered as "normal" up to a certain point. It is this point that keeps getting pushed higher and higher, extending the limits of "normal" to include more people. If all the policemen in the United States with more than five years of service had to take a hearing examination under present regulations, the majority would fail due to exposure to gunfire alone.

PRESBYCUSIS (HEARING LOSS WITH AGE)

Aging is an inevitable process we all must face with advancing years. The skin wrinkles. Hair thins. Bones ache.

And in this change, many people develop high frequency sensorineural hearing losses referred to as presbycusis.

Actually, hearing loss in the higher frequencies begins after birth and deterioration continues throughout life. Newborns with normal hearing hear up to as high as 20,000 Hz. A young adult may not be able to hear beyond 16,000 Hz, and by the age of 80, most people cannot hear above 6,000 Hz.

Presbycusis generally appears as noticeable to an individual after the age of 40, and more often in men than women. The loss is bilaterally symmetrical (occurring in both ears to the same degree) and may progress at varying rates throughout life. Tinnitus (ringing in the ears) and vertigo have been associated with presbycusis. In one study of more than 500 presbycusic individuals, 50 percent reported tinnitus and about a third reported vertigo.

The cause of presbycusis is unknown (although there is serious speculation) and there is no successful medical treatment for it. A frequently used explanation for presbycusis is arteriosclerosis or atherosclerosis (see "Diet-Hearing-Coronary Heart Disease," p. 62). There is clinical evidence indicating that such vascular changes do occur in many presbycusic ears.

Long-term noise exposure and presbycusis frequently reveal identical configurations on the audiogram. What has been referred to for years as "presbycusis" may be little more than hearing loss from noise (or diet). In many senior citizens with presbycusis, exposure to noise has been denied, yet there is still the possibility that such people simply did not consider what they were exposed to as dangerously loud noise. If a bus speeds past you at 50 mph and thrusts out 95 dB of noise, you may not consider it as harmful, but as normal! The fact is, such noise may contribute to permanent hearing loss.

The case of "presbycusis" and "noise-induced hearing loss" being one and the same in terms of causes is strongly supported by one investigator who studied a primitive culture in Africa that had not been exposed to noise nor even loud singing. Results of the investigation of hearing in the elders revealed that nobody suffered from presbycusis to the degree that people in "civilized" societies do. Furthermore, when some

51

natives moved from their remote region of Africa to the hustle and bustle of city life, within a matter of years they developed presbycusis, as well as arteriosclerosis and heart disease! Many factors that were not controlled may have produced hearing deterioration (such as diet, genetics, climate, etc.) but environmental noise *must* be considered as the strongest contender. What has been considered as acceptable environmental noise may well indeed be extremely detrimental to our hearing.[66]

The elderly have been the ones exposed the longest to environmental noise pollution. It seems only too obvious that what we have been referring to as "presbycusis—cause unknown" with many patients appears to be long-term exposure to environmental noise.

THE FUTURE

We have slowly grown accustomed to a level of noise in our environment that now *must* be considered dangerous. High level noise emissions persist and are getting louder. Many people mistakenly believe that the more noise you can tolerate, the stronger you are. Still others mistakenly equate noise with productivity. A great many industrial and construction workers do not utilize ear protection when it can be effective. And we tend to think that if a particular product we buy makes a lot of noise, then it must be made very well. But the absence of noise does not necessarily mean a reduction in productivity!

A lawn mower manufacturer produced a new mower recently that was marketed as the quietest model of its kind. Those who purchased the mower complained after using it that it was not as powerful as their older machines (meaning the noisier ones). But this new lawn mower was in fact as powerful as other competitive models. The company had great difficulty selling these substantially quieter machines. Noise has become equated with power and production. This is not a new phenomenon. As I said at the beginning of this chapter, it probably started with the Industrial Revolution and all the new inventions of machinery in the 1700's. If we are to fight the battle against noise, and win, we must first recognize our enemy s being noise.

Many scientists are now realizing that exposure to noise levels in excess of 70 dB may be detrimental to our health. The frightening thing here is that our environmental noise level on any given day is approximately 70 dB. More alarming yet is that the average noise level within our homes is now considered to be approximately 70 dB and, like environmental noise, it is increasing.

The end result of all these years of noise is not going to be visible "someday." We are there. It has already happened! Noise can cause hearing loss. Unfortunately, with space age technology, things are not getting quieter. And space age technology is only beginning.

We all contribute to the noise problem. We drive cars, own barking dogs, use tools, shoot cap guns to cannons, and utilize the convenience of electrical devices from air conditioners to hair blowers.

To avoid potential hearing damage, we must avoid those products that produce excessive noise. Even writing the manufacturers of such companies can have a tremendous positive effect, informing them that you are aware of and bothered by this by-product (see Appendix III).

We generally never need music or television as loud as it is. And if discotheque or movie theater sound levels are too loud, report it to the owner! Become more aware of the intensities that you are exposed to and have been putting up with without knowing it for your entire life.

The medicolegal problems now surfacing from years of noise exposure to many employees are making employers more aware and concerned about this problem. Unfortunately, most employers are not concerned with the potential hearing problem that can result from noise exposure; they are concerned with the potential legal ramifications.

Attorneys are now realizing the grand profits that exist in handling cases of noise-induced hearing loss. This is bound to get more attention in the future, as noise not only persists, but gets louder. We are heading toward another medicolegal crisis similar to the malpractice crisis that physicians faced only a short time ago.

In the past 20 years, the loudest noises to which man has been exposed have been getting louder by one decibel per years. We could say that in 20 more years, if noise is allowed to increase, the problem will be out of control. But the fact is that noise is out of control NOW!

"Sociocusis" is a hearing loss attributable to environmental noise. We will become more and more familiar with this term in the future and, if in fact noise is allowed to increase at the steady rate it has been for the past 20 years, we can expect that nobody will have "normal" hearing, as we now know it, over the age of 10 by the year 2000.

Chapter IV
TYPES OF
HEARING DISORDERS

PART I: CAUSES AND TREATMENTS

There are two basic types of hearing loss: 1) conductive and 2) sensorineural. A combination of both is referred to as a mixed loss. Treatment exists for conductive impairments through surgical procedures, frequently with very successful results. However, for sensorineural hearing loss, no surgical treatment is available that has been established and recognized for this condition. The control of sensorineural problems has been far more successful in terms of prevention than cure.

A conductive hearing loss is a hearing loss that exists as a result of some mechanical difficulty in the conduction of sound through the middle ear. Although there can be conductive problems within the cochlea, I am speaking of surgically reparable problems. Surgical results on conductive impairments are generally quite good with more than 90 percent of all conductive impairments responding favorably.

Assuming that the hearing problem is a purely conductive one, the problem is being unable to receive voices loud enough. If speech sounds are made loud enough, there is no problem in understanding what is said. People with conductive hearing loss find that they actually hear better in noisy places, quite unlike people with sensorineural loss. Since the conductive hearing loss is one that can be compensated for if sound is made loud enough, there is little difficulty in noisy situations. Background noise doesn't bother the person with conductive impairment because he can't hear these background noises very well anyway. And since normal hearing persons exposed to the same noises hear the background noises quite loud, they raise their voices above the level of ambient noise so as to hear one another better. In so doing, their voices are loud enough for the conductive impaired person to hear well also.

The most common cause of conductive hearing loss is fluid in the middle ears (otitis media). Another very common cause is otosclerosis. Both will be discussed in part two of this chapter.

The individual with a sensorineural hearing loss suffers from an abnormality of the sense organ, auditory nerve or both. Many people with sensorineural hearing loss find that even if sound is made loud enough, it is not clear and easy to distinguish. This difficulty is greatly increased in the presence of background noise. The greater the hearing loss and the intensity of the background noise, the greater the difficulty in understanding for the sensorineurally impaired individual.

Sensorineural hearing loss is the condition that most people with a hearing loss suffer from. It is estimated that more than 33 million people in the United States experience sensorineural impairment great enough to impair communications.

For the millions of people with sensorineural hearing loss—attributable to noise exposure, head traumas, medication, aging, polio, smallpox, chicken pox, mumps, measles, rubella, herpes simplex, respiratory viruses, scarlet fever, infectious hepatitis or mononucleosis, meningitis, influenza, common cold, pneumonia or infection in the ear—there is no surgical restoration. Usually the damage is permanent. However, in some instances, the hearing has been known to return without any treatment whatsoever.

Indirectly, hearing has been altered through intravenous treatments in such cases as very sudden hearing loss, diabetes, Meniere's Disorder and other unusual conditions where hearing is the apparent symptom of a yet more serious condition. One day perhaps cochlear transplants may become as frequent a surgical procedure as kidney, lung or heart transplants. But presently, cochlear transplants are only at a theoretical level of development.

HEAD BLOWS

Head blows have been shown to cause serious high frequency hearing loss. Contact sports such as football, rugby, wrestling, and in particular, boxing, can cause hearing loss. Since the damage is in the higher range, it is usually the "quality" of speech that is affected, and because quality is so subjective, it often goes undetected for years until the loss is quite pronounced.

Head blows have been studied on rats, guinea pigs, cats, dogs and humans. All such studies (except the human studies) required beating the skulls with a weapon. An audiogram revealed high frequency hearing loss. This was confirmed upon removal of the inner ear. Dissection indicated inner ear hemorrhages in many of these animals, causing the hearing loss.[67-69]

In 1969, a case was reported of a woman who fell down a flight of stairs, struck her head, went into a coma and died from central nervous system injuries. A postmortem examination of the inner ears revealed that hearing impairment was present in the higher ranges due to the accident.[70] It is also not unusual to discover hearing loss as the result of an auto accident. Head trauma can be lethal to the hearing mechanism.

CERUMEN (EARWAX)

No surgical procedure exists for removing wax in the ear. It is generally removed without difficulty or complications by an ear wash or irrigation (with a syringe). Sometimes a solution is used to soften it before it is removed. In cases where the wax is hardened, a physician can often pull it out with the proper instrument.

Cerumen is formed by the secretion of two glands. The rate of production seems to vary from person to person, and personal hygiene often determines how much wax collects in the outer ear canal. Some researchers believe that wax is removed from the canal through jaw movement such as chewing or talking.

The determining factors of earwax production are really not well understood. Some researchers believe it to be affected by the same variables that exist for perspiration, but others discount this theory.

Even less understood than production is the purpose of earwax. There are some interesting suggestions but none can actually be held as the primary purpose. Some generally accepted purposes presented by scientists in the past are that wax helps in the removal of epidermal scales in the canal; prevents the canal from drying out; or deters insects from getting too close to the eardrum by its adhesive quality (although recent research evidence indicates that earwax does not repel insects whatsoever).

The color of cerumen depends upon its age. Wax can range from yellow to black and from very soft to very hard consistency. Fresh earwax is usually yellow and soft while older cerumen is often brown or darker in color and much harder.

Histochemical studies on cerumen have shown that it is made of elements including: calcium, chloride, cholesterol, hydrogen, magnesium, phosphorus, potassium, silicon, sodium, sulfur, as well as cerotic acid, neostearic acid and many amino acids.

For some people, overproduction of cerumen can create problems that range from itching to hearing loss. However, in cases of excessive amounts of wax that do cause hearing loss, the impairment is temporary if the wax is removed promptly. Occasionally, cerumen can build up against the eardrum causing severe pain, in addition to hearing loss. But this occurs in people who either have an excessive production of wax, neglect removing it, or impact it into the canal when trying to remove it with a cotton swab or other probe.

EARWAX REMOVAL

Since wax production is a normal bodily function, it isn't something we would want to stop, or for that matter, might be able to stop. Wax production occurs much like perspiration. The question is not one of how to stop it, but how to control it.

Nobody can overemphasize how dangerous it is to use cotton-tipped swabs for the removal of cerumen. Such probing can rub away protective layers of keratin, leaving skin cells exposed to possible infection. There is an even greater chance that the cotton swab could be pushed through the eardrum causing problems that may range from severe pain to total deafness in the traumatized ear. Often-reported objects used by people to remove cerumen include sticks, rat-tailed combs, hair pins, bobby pins, pens, plastic forks and paper clips—all of which can produce serious injury.

Very often, cotton swabs push wax further into the ear canal, eventually producing an impaction of wax. It's not unusual for mothers to use cotton swabs to clean their infants' ears. Their intentions are good, but they don't realize that this is not necessary and can produce complications. An estimated one-half million children a year are seen by physicians due to impacted wax from the use of cotton swabs.[71]

The ear needs nothing more than soap and water and a wash cloth to be kept clean. Any medicinal applications such as drops or ointment should be used *only* upon the recommendation *and* prescription of a physician.

TINNITUS (RINGING)

Ringing in the ears is one of the most common complaints of people with or without hearing loss. The condition is called tinnitus. In some cases, it may be a warning sign that damage has occurred to the hearing mechanism and to be aware of future abuses. An estimated 86 percent of patients seen by audiologists and otologists complain of tinnitus. Also, it is reported more often in individuals over the age of 40.[72]

There are generally two types of tinnitus: 1) objective and 2) subjective. Objective tinnitus, under certain conditions, can be heard by an observer. That is, due to some unusual vascular or muscular phenomenon,[73] there is either a clicking or squeaking that is actually emitted from the ear and can be heard if you (as the observer) listen for it close to the ear.

Much more common is subjective tinnitus, which is only audible to the individual complaining of it. Subjective tinnitus can be caused by anything from wax in the ear to some neurological phenomenon between the ear and the brain. The possibilities of a problem occurring somewhere along the path between the ear and brain that could produce tinnitus are considerable. This includes the middle ear cavity where fluid can build up and produce ringing or where a malfunction of any of the tiny bones, muscles or eustachian tube can occur.[74,75] But even more often, subjective tinnitus is suspected to be caused somewhere within the neurological system.

In most instances, authorities report that tinnitus probably occurs as the result of some chemical or electrical disturbance somewhere between the cochlea and the brain. The ringing in such cases is reported as being high-pitched, and has been described as sounding like bells, humming, buzzing, hissing, escaping steam, whistling, roaring, or sounds of ocean waves. In the more infrequent complaints when the tinnitus is associated with the outer or middle ear, it is reported as being low-pitched, and has been described as a ticking, clicking, snapping, popping or crackling. The ringing may be long or short in duration, in one or both ears, and sometimes changing in pitch. It may be constant, aperiodic, or even pulsating (seemingly with the heartbeat).

Worrying that you are losing your hearing, going deaf or growing a tumor is unwarranted, although these fears are common among people who suffer from tinnitus. Many people without any hearing loss whatsoever experience bothersome ringing at times. In fact, one researcher carried out a study on the effects of silence on normal hearing individuals. One hundred such listeners (all with normal hearing) were evaluated in a sound-treated room under identical conditions. The results were then compared to 100 hearing impaired individuals to see the effect of silence on hearing. Results showed that 73 percent of the hard of hearing group reported hearing some kind of ringing in their ears while experiencing the silence. Ninety-four percent of the normal hearing group reported the same. So, although tinnitus may be a symptom of hearing difficulty or potential problems, it often is found in people with no hearing deficit at all.

It has been suggested that excess amounts of alcohol, tobacco, coffee, tea, or aspirin could cause or aggravate the condition. Tinnitus has been associated with exposure to intense noise, changes in air pressure, headaches, fatigue, nervous tension and general illness. Emotions have been suggested as a cause of tinnitus, affecting inner ear fluids or blood supply to the inner ear.[76] In such cases, the louder the ringing, the greater the anxiety which may in turn increase the tinnitus which increases the anxiety, continuing in an endless cycle. Tinnitus has never been known to drive anyone crazy— although at times it seems to. It has been bothersome enough to many people to such a point that they develop excess tension, irritability, frustration or any of a number of other emotional or neurotic conditions.

Many people complain that their ringing is so loud that they cannot fall asleep at night. For my patients who complain of this, I recommend that they put a radio near their bed and put on some very soft background music. Many have found this remedy to work well for them since the soft music masks the ringing in the ears. But for some, the music is as disturbing as the tinnitus.

Surgical treatment has been used in handling tinnitus but without dependable results. In the millions of people with tinnitus produced by some anomaly between the cochlea and the brain, there has been no documented, successful treatment, particularly when the tinnitus has been a long-standing problem. Otologists have used vasodilation (such as treatment with nicotinic acid), but unfortunately, with disappointing results. Other medications have been tried and as yet there is no real treatment. Dietary control has been tried with some qualified success.

Although we have been successful in the discovery of planets billions of miles apart, and have been able to man space vehicles for hundreds of thousands of miles into the outer reaches of space, scientists are still studying the causes of and cures for tinnitus that travels only inches between the ear and the brain.

DIET—HEARING—CORONARY HEART DISEASE

A definite relationship exists between what we eat, how we feel and how long we live. There are more people affected by coronary heart disease today than ever before. The American Heart Association reported in 1976 that an estimated 28,830,000 people suffer from serious heart disease in the United States. It is the single most frequent cause of death in this country, and it is increasing.

Extensive research has been carried out in the area of diet and heart disease. What has been discovered from hundreds of studies is a definite correlation between saturated fats, high serum cholesterol levels in the blood and coronary heart disease.

The 1960's was a period with much attention focused on diet and saturated fats. Many food manufacturers jumped on the bandwagon and produced highly unsaturated fat products. Low-fat, non-fat and skim milk products quickly became popular substitutes. Margarine replaced butter and supposedly reduced the **chances** of developing coronary heart disease. Eggs were found to be cholesterol producing and were recommended to be greatly reduced in the diet.

But the fact is that there is no evidence that any replacement of saturated fats in our diet with unsaturated fats (e.g., replacing whole milk and butter with non-fat milk and margarine) will reduce **the chances of** heart disease.[77] This is supported by numerous studies, many on rhesus monkeys, whereby high cholesterol levels and high saturated fat diets resulted in fatal heart attacks.[78] Further investigation has shown that atherosclerosis (a degeneration of the walls of the heart, resulting in heart disease) has been reversed in the rhesus monkey when put on a low-fat/low-cholesterol diet, *instead of* replacing saturated fats with unsaturated fats.[79,80] This was further substantiated in a study on 200 men with a history of heart attacks who were put on a diet that replaced their saturated fats with unsaturated fats. Results of this study revealed that these known heart attack victims were no safer with unsaturated fats, because their incidence of heart disease remained the same after being on the diet. Their death rate as compared to the control group was not different.[81]

Additional support is observed in other human studies that are quite impressive. Two separate primitive African tribes (the Bantus and the Mabaans) were studied by separate investigators.[82-84] Both groups were found to have a very low-fat/low-cholesterol existence. Coronary heart disease in both groups was literally non-existent.

Hence, what researchers have found is that a low-fat/low-cholesterol diet decreases the chances of coronary heart disease and that replacing saturated fats with unsaturated fats seems to have no effect.

We establish our diet of high or low cholesterol when we are very young. We generally fall into the diet that our parents establish for us. If parents are on a high-fat diet, generally their children will be also. Hence, if children remain on high saturated fat diets, we would expect them to develop heart disease. And they do. Research reveals that heart disease begins when we are very young. However, it takes many years on the diet before its true deleterious effects are visible. Nonetheless, research evidence exists to show that children and young adults under the age of 21 have very definite signs of heart disease.[85,86]

If the heart is affected, then we would expect that whatever organs that the heart pumps blood to would also be affected. The inner ear depends upon a constant fresh flow of blood for the nutrients that keep it functioning. Since the source of this blood is the heart, any damage to the heart might well affect the flow, quantity, or quality of blood to the inner ear. So if the arteries are clogged and blood circulation is impaired, it is conceivable that hearing loss could be a secondary effect of heart disease. Research studies support this possibility.

A long-term study was begun on two groups of patients in a part of the world with the highest saturated fats in the diet, highest serum cholesterol levels and the highest incidence of coronary heart disease. The study took place in Finland.[87]

Group A was allowed to maintain their extremely high-fat/high-cholesterol diet for five years and was observed and evaluated closely. Group B was taken off the high-fat/high-cholesterol diet and was put on a low-fat/low-cholesterol diet and also followed closely for five years. Results included the following: 1) the serum cholesterol levels in the blood of Group A (high-fat diet) had not changed while in Group B, the levels had dropped dramatically; 2) Group B increased their blood coagulability time (observed within six months after the start of the study) while Group A's did not change; 3) the incidence of coronary heart disease was higher in Group A than in Group B; 4) hearing evaluations revealed that the hearing acuity of Group B was superior *at all frequencies tested* to Group A. In fact, patients in Group B heard better than a matched number of patients *ten years younger* in Group A!

For further validation, the researchers reversed the diets of the two groups to see if the results would then also reverse. So Group A (high-fat diet) was put on a low-fat/low-cholesterol diet while Group B (formerly low-fat diet) was put back on their original high-fat diet.[88,89]

The results after three and a half years proved what was expected: the now high-fat diet group no longer had better hearing acuity, but the low-fat diet group (formerly on the high-fat diet) had improved hearing. The reversal in the diet therefore also reversed a progression in hearing loss.

The possible conclusions that can be drawn from this study are phenomenal. Not only can a low-fat/low-cholesterol diet prevent loss of hearing, but it may well reverse the loss and improve hearing. The losses studied were of the sensorineural type.

The life support system for the ear is blood that comes from the heart. An impairment to this circulatory system *can* impair hearing. However, the loss of hearing is actually a secondary effect of a much greater problem—coronary heart disease. Hence, it may be entirely possible to predict coronary heart disease by observable signs of a change in hearing.

Much more extensive investigation into this area of study is badly needed. It is certainly warranted in the light of present knowledge.

DRUGS AND HEARING

The combination of various medications within the body may act to produce hearing problems, but if consumed independently may not be harmful. Pharmacologists admit their naivete in unfolding the mysteries behind the apparent curing effects of many drugs. Physicians prescribe drugs because they bring about a desired effect, although *how* that effect is brought about is often a mystery. Drug interaction has been studied by clinical pharmacists in many large hospitals throughout the United States. It has been generally agreed that the hair cells of the inner ear are the primary target of ototoxicity (hearing loss due to medication), while nerve degeneration is secondary.[90]

ALCOHOL, TOBACCO, COFFEE AND ASPIRIN

Excessive amounts of alcohol, tobacco, caffeine, aspirin and tonic water can cause or aggravate hearing impairment.

Alcohol is a known ototoxic drug. It is not uncommon to find hearing loss in heavy drinkers, in addition to complaints of tinnitus. Considering that an estimated 100 million people in the United States "drink" and that Alcoholics Anonymous report 10 million American alcoholics, it is amazing that the hearing problems that alcohol can produce have not been reported in greater numbers in the past.

Nicotine is a known vasoconstrictor. It inhibits the flow of blood throughout the body by narrowing the blood vessels—including those nourishing the ear. It can cause ringing in the ears as well as hearing loss. Various research data even reveals that nonsmokers respond far more favorably to surgery than smokers of at least one pack per day. Ear surgery such as reconstruction of a new eardrum (myringoplasty), one of the least dangerous and complex operations of the ear, has statistically higher failure rates among people who smoke (20+ cigarettes per day).[91] Realizing that an estimated 50 million Americans presently smoke at least a pack a day and that billions of cigarettes are manufactured each year, it is almost certain that we have only begun to recognize the relationship between nicotine and hearing loss. The fact is that the death

65

rate from heart disease is 70 percent higher among smokers than nonsmokers.[92] Since the heart pumps blood through the inner ear, supplying it with necessary nutrients, if degenerative disease occurs in the heart, inner ear blood flow can be affected resulting in potential hearing loss.

And what American household does not contain a coffee pot? The vast quantity of coffee that is consumed annually in the United States alone is in excess of every man, woman and child drinking one cup *every* day. More coffee beans were marketed in the recent past than ever before. The number of cups of coffee that could be poured from this past year's harvest are in the trillions of cups. This does not include tea, which contains just as much caffeine. Both are central nervous system stimulants. Caffeine has been *positively* correlated with frequency of heart disease.[93] Caffeine has been proven to increase the serum cholesterol level which leads to heart disease.[94] A secondary effect of high caffeine intake is tinnitus, often described as loud and long-lasting ringing. Many of my patients who have complained of tinnitus and also drink excessive amounts of coffee have been amazed to discover that with a reduction in their caffeine intake, their tinnitus has decreased. But this is assuming that the caffeine was the cause in the first place.

Nearly one million people die each year from heart disease. The number of people who suffer from tinnitus or hearing loss as a result of their heart disease is impossible to calculate. Research in this area is nonexistent. Someday, it may well be discovered that tinnitus and/or hearing loss *may* be an indicator of approaching heart disease.

Aspirin consumption in the United States has reached an alarming level. Americans consume more aspirin than any other country. The Department of Commerce reported that 31,668,000 pounds—equivalent to *thirty-five and one-half billion tablets*—were consumed in 1971! The exact way in which aspirin affects hearing is not fully understood. However, the effects themselves are understood, at least in part—aspirin causes tinnitus and hearing loss in many people who ingest it. It usually takes large dosages to produce these effects, but this is not to suggest that small dosages do not carry the same effects. They may, only less intensely (see case history nine, p. 151).

The actual effects of any of the aforementioned ingestables are extremely difficult to evaluate. The effects are insidious: slow to occur, slow to be recognized and frequently overlooked as being the cause of any of the symptoms discussed.

The frequent warning signs from the effects of alcohol, nicotine, caffeine and aspirin include: headaches, dizziness, vertigo, tinnitus, loss of balance or pressure around the ears (or fullness in the ears). All of these may also be signs of potential hearing loss. Awareness of these facts is imperative and caution as to the intake of these chemicals is a must if we are to eliminate the threat that they pose to our systems.

DRUGS AND PREGNANCY

A dangerous period for a pregnant woman to ingest any medication is during the first trimester of pregnancy. This is a time when the fetus is most vulnerable to environmental factors such as infection, toxins or drugs. Many physicians request pregnant women to abstain from tobacco, alcohol and coffee for this reason. During the first three months of fetal growth, the inner ear develops rapidly. A mother stricken with measles (rubella) during this period has statistically higher odds of producing an offspring with hearing defects. These odds drop dramatically by the fourth month, at which time formation of the inner ear is complete.

Medical research also indicates that the oral contraceptive pill for women may lead to tinnitus, vertigo, and hearing loss. Such inner ear pathology would certainly warrant more extensive investigation.[95]

QUININE AND SULFA DRUGS

During World War I, veterans were treated heavily with quinine and sulfa drugs to combat widespread malaria. The drugs have been devastating to thousands of veterans because of their harmful effects on hearing. Any chemical agents that get into the blood have the potential for altering the state of hearing. The tiny hair cells in the cochlea can be permanently damaged. The Veterans Administration compensates hundreds of thousands of veterans for hearing loss, many caused by such chemical agents. (See Appendix II for list of known drugs associated with hearing damage.)

ANTIBIOTICS

A common group of pharmacological agents includes the mycins, such as streptomycin, an antibiotic frequently prescribed for control of a wide range of conditions. One of hundreds of medical reports on the mycins revealed that small doses of injected streptomycin produce convulsions in rabbits, followed by respiratory paralysis and death.

The pharmacology of one particular antibiotic used in medical treatment of the ear was reviewed in *Science Digest*, January 1975. It revealed that chloramphenicol (Chloromycetin) has been the cause of death in hundreds of documented cases. It has been used for anything from the common cold with sniffles to the crippling condition of meningitis.

In 1969, a medical report stated that a four-year-old boy had been treated for recurrent meningitis, associated with a head trauma from an auto accident one year earlier. The child was treated for more than a year when finally he underwent major ear surgery. The child appeared well for about 18 months when once again he was admitted to the hospital with meningitis. The child was admitted in poor condition and died after massive intravenous doses of chloramphenicol (and other medication). An attempt to save a child's life may actually have killed him. The first warnings of chloramphenicol's potential deleterious effects reached the news media in the 1940's. However, the drug is still widely used today. In fact, it is prescribed about 20 times as often as is actually necessary.

MIRACLE CURES?

There have been many widely publicized sure-cure remedies to nerve-type hearing loss, nearly all of which have no scientific evidence to support their claims of "miracle cures." But such campaigns continue causing hearing impaired people financial and emotional problems. Perhaps one day far into the future we will be able to wake up and pop a pill for breakfast and know we have all the minimum daily nutritional requirements. Perhaps then there may even be a machine we would stand before that could reveal any physical disorders of the body, for which there would be a "pink pill" to bring about an immediate cure. But until these miracles are discovered, the inadequacies of the 20th century will have to be endured. There are no such miracle cures yet for hearing disorders.

FLUORIDE

Fluoride has been thought of primarily in terms of reducing tooth decay. It is believed to strengthen the bones of the body as well. Not too ironically, the strongest bone in the body is the cochlea (mechanism for hearing) located in the inner ear that houses the delicate parts for sound reception. Research has revealed that tooth decay occurs less in those areas of the United States where fluoride content in water is high. Otosclerosis (a softening of bone within the middle or inner ear) has also been shown to occur less in those same parts of the country. Hence, it appears that fluoride not only helps in preventing tooth decay, but may actually help to prevent otosclerosis. If a hearing problem is already present, though, no amount of fluoride treatments seems to have any effect.

VITAMINS

As early as the 19th century it was believed that certain vitamins could prevent or cure deafness or hearing loss. Vitamin A was given in massive doses in the treatment of sensorineural deafness, but was ineffective. Recently and only in certain rare cases, vitamin A has appeared to have some positive effect on hearing where nerve deafness is not the primary problem. There is some reported qualified success in the treatment of Meniere's Disorder and in a few other instances where the loss was sudden. However, optimism must be restrained until further research sheds more light.

In 1947, 3,667 prisoners of war returned to the United States with multiple deficiencies of B vitamins. Thirteen of the

prisoners had nerve-type deafness and some physicians correlated the lack of B vitamins with the nerve impairment. This
association has not been substantiated by scientific evidence.
Several of the B vitamins are necessary for the maintenance of
normal central nervous system functioning, but if vitamin
deficiency is indeed a causative factor in deafness, once the
deprivation has occurred there is no evidence that massive
treatments of any vitamin can restore proper hearing.[96]

EAR MASSAGE

There is absolutely no truth in the claim that an ear
massage can restore hearing in a clinically diagnosed case of
nerve deafness. Despite this fact, in some cases of sensorineural
hearing loss, people have insisted that they hear better if they
press on the skull behind the ear, or tilt the head, or apply
pressure to the neck. There is no scientific explanation for such
phenomena. When there is a problem with the eustachian tube
(a middle ear condition) hearing actually *can* be restored in
some cases through gentle massage. This is unrelated to nerve
impairment and is not a recommended procedure for resolving
one's hearing disorder. In such cases, the eustachian tube does
not function to equalize pressure in the middle ear cavity, and
therefore rubbing the ear gently, yawning, swallowing, chewing, rotating the jaw, or holding the nose closed while trying to
blow through it can fill the middle ear with the needed air.
Altitudinal changes exemplify this condition. However, ear
massage can result in disarticulation of the middle ear bones
(malleus, incus or stapes) and can be dangerous.

EARDROPS

Eardrops are prescribed for certain conditions of the outer
or middle ear but they do not affect, nor are they intended to
affect the inner ear. There is no truth in the statement that
eardrops can restore hearing in cases of neural damage.
However, they may help in the treatment of itching, discomfort, or infection of the outer or middle ear cavities. Eardrops
should only be used upon the recommendation of your physician.

NEURAL IMPLANTS

Neural implants are a rather recent procedure. An electrical device is placed in the inner ear allowing reception of very gross sounds. So far, it has only been used in cases of profound deafness where no hearing was present in either ear. The implants are presently of no value to the hard of hearing person but may someday replace hearing aids for people with defective hearing. That day is not within sight yet.

STAPLEPUNCTURE

Some physicians have used staples in the earlobes or other parts of the outer ear to produce weight reduction in their patients. The physicians report that their patients merely touch the metal staple(s) and their desire for eating disappears. A miracle! The procedure is known as staplepuncture and only works in cases where the patients are prone to suggestion. The weight reduction is totally unrelated to either the ear, the hearing, or the touching of the metal implant—other than the fact that there is an obvious psychological effect at work if one *believes* that touching this metal staple will cause loss of appetite. There is a very high risk of developing an ear infection and therefore the staples are frequently removed shortly after insertion. For this reason, according to otologists, the procedure must be considered dangerous.

ACUPUNCTURE

Acupuncture for hearing restoration has received much attention in recent years and has been the subject of considerable controversy. There is no scientific evidence that it has any effect upon hearing, positive or negative. A leading corporation in the U.S. launched a research project on the success-failure rate of acupuncture.[97] Questionnaires were sent to major university and community speech and hearing centers around the U.S., as well as to community hospitals, university hospitals, the Veterans Administration hospitals, aural rehabilitation centers, schools for the deaf, public schools for the hearing impaired, state programs for cerebral palsy and mental retardation, and to clinical audiologists in private practice. There were over 300 responses, with no significant indications that acupuncture had been successful in the treatment of sensorineural hearing impairment.

There are isolated documented reports of remarkable changes in hearing, but the variables involved are too great to attribute acupuncture as the causative factor in hearing alteration. Some people suffer from fluctuant hearing loss due to a vascular disorder. Also, a change in hearing threshold occurs during and after exposure to loud noise. Hence, if a patient goes in for acupuncture treatment on a day of poor hearing and the ear recovers naturally, it might be concluded that the treatment produced an increase in hearing. Such results would be erroneous to say the least.

Acupuncture is still in the primitive stages and its relation to hearing is as yet unfounded. The principle of acupuncture is based upon the Chinese life forces of "Yin" and "Yang" and it is believed that these forces can rejuvenate deteriorated or dead tissue in the inner ear as it relates to hearing. Scientifically, such an explanation is unsubstantiated. Once the hair cells of the inner ear have degenerated, they cannot produce new growth, unlike some other follicles in the human body. There is a very strong psychological element in acupuncture—after having paid anywhere from a few hundred dollars to a few thousand dollars for treatments, certainly it would be hoped or expected that hearing would be improved. Many physicians have referred to it as "quackupuncture." Until the Nobel Prize has been given for such a breakthrough, acupuncture for hearing must be considered purely experimental with recently reported findings discouraging. Such claims as having a 90 percent cure-rate* in China, or a 10 percent cure-rate in the U.S., are simply unfounded (see case history eight, p. 148).

SOUND ADVICE

Suffice it to say that there are many myths that still exist concerning the medicinal and non-medical miracle cures for

---

*More recently, reports from China have claimed 8 to 11 percent, but still remain completely undocumented.

hearing impairment. The most acceptable "cure" to hearing impairment is through surgery.

PART II: EAR SURGERY

Certain kinds of hearing losses respond quite favorably to ear surgery. These are primarily conductive hearing difficulties where a mechanical problem exists, preventing proper transmission of sound beyond the middle ear cavity. Better than 90 percent of such types of hearing losses can benefit from surgery. Sensorineural hearing losses are operable only in very rare cases and usually with poor results.

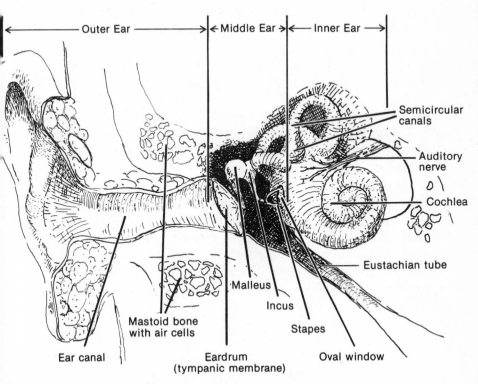

Figure 4: The parts of the ear.

This part of the chapter focuses on conductive losses and the surgical procedures involved, as well as the preoperative and postoperative results on hearing. Recent research data and clinical findings have also been included to provide you with an up-to-date perspective on surgery as it relates to hearing.

Ear surgery may involve some risks that include a decrease or loss in sensation, dizziness, hypersensitivity to sounds, facial paralysis, and/or partial or complete loss of hearing. There are always risks when undergoing any surgery even with the best surgeons, so it's advisable to seek out the most competent surgeon available. At least one outside medical opinion about the procedure should be obtained from another medical source.

ACUTE AND CHRONIC OTITIS MEDIA

A major health concern for many parents is fluid (otitis media) in the ears of their children. It is a condition often found in people with a simple common cold, and frequently found in children under ten years of age. There are several different kinds of otitis media, most of which are accompanied by hearing loss in advanced stages of the infection. The problem is in the middle ear cavity where mechanical action of the ossicles (malleus, incus, stapes) is reduced due to the fluid.

Acute otitis media usually occurs bilaterally and is often the result of upper respiratory infection, allergies, sinusitis, hypertrophied adenoids, improper nose blowing, sneezing, or eustachian tube blockage. The condition is considered acute as long as the ear responds to treatment. If it recurs, even time and time again, followed by temporary successful medical treatment, the ear suffers from recurrent acute otitis media. However, if the infection persists without responding to treatment after one or two months, the condition is considered to be chronic. In either acute or chronic otitis media, serious hearing impairment can result. The hearing loss, although most often of a temporary nature, can lead to permanent sensorineural impairment if left untreated.

In one study, over 400 patients with diagnosed chronic otitis media were followed for a five-year period from 1964 to

1969.[98] The results indicated that permanent sensorineural hearing loss can result. The investigators came to this conclusion after finding that the more severe the infection and the greater the duration of the infection, the greater the likelihood of some permanent sensorineural hearing loss. For this reason, otologists try to find immediate relief from the infection and/or pain. Some otologists perform surgery to treat the infection, while other otologists prefer the use of antibiotics and attempt surgery only when absolutely indicated.

MYRINGOTOMY

The surgical procedure for removal of fluid from the middle ear cavity is a myringotomy. The procedure involves a surgical incision in the eardrum allowing the fluid to drain out. Statistically, the ear has less chance of permanent damage and complications if the hole in the drum is surgically performed. People who neglect the problem often experience a sudden rupture in the eardrum as a result of fluid pressure built up in the middle ear cavity. If pus is trapped in the middle ear causing the eardrum to bulge, a myringotomy is often performed to prevent hearing loss and relieve pain. In cases of chronic middle ear infection, a tube is often inserted into the eardrum to allow fluid to drain continually. The tube may remain in place from within six months to as long as two years, providing aeration of the middle ear cavity in an attempt to avoid reaccumulation of secretions.

There has been much investigation into and controversy over the effects of myringotomies in children (and adults).[99] Research has turned up significant evidence to indicate that myringotomies cause tympanosclerosis (scarred drums and bony deposits around the stapes frequently making it less mobile).[100] Also, evidence indicates that greater hearing loss exists in children who develop tympanosclerosis (as a result of tube insertion) following myringotomy compared to children who never had tubes inserted following myringotomies.[101] The incidence appears to have a rather wide range. However, approximately 30 percent of children in various studies who have undergone myringotomies with tubes have developed tympanosclerosis, according to recent reports by many investigators. Because of these risks, such techniques deserve closer scrutiny.

MYRINGOPLASTY

An eardrum may be totally or partially missing as the result of a birth deformity, a trauma or infection. The method of closing a perforation in an eardrum is myringoplasty. This is done only in the absence of infection. One research study indicates that better than 99 percent of such procedures have been successful at a major ear clinic in Los Angeles. Audiologically, hearing has been completely restored through this grafting process. If a hearing loss does persist following myringoplasty, and the operation was successful, then it is likely that some other problem is producing the impairment.[102]

TYMPANOPLASTY
(MODIFIED RADICAL MASTOIDECTOMY)

An infection in the middle ear cavity can produce serious hearing loss as a result of erosion of the ossicles and/or the eardrum. In such cases, the surgeon's objective is to remove the diseased tissue and reconstruct any of the destroyed mechanical parts. This operation is known as tympanoplasty. A number of factors must be considered in the prognosis of postoperative hearing: age of patient, any current drainage from the ear, previous ear disease, degree of hearing impairment prior to surgery, and the type of tympanoplasty planned.[103,104]

SIMPLE AND RADICAL MASTOIDECTOMY

When acute otitis media has infected the mastoid air cells, a simple mastoidectomy may be performed, often with no loss in hearing. The purpose is to eradicate the mastoid bone of all diseased tissue. The operation allows drainage of secretions that could otherwise dangerously build up within the middle ear cavity. It usually leaves a scar just behind the flap of the outer ear. This procedure is rarely performed today due to improved management of otitis media.

Radical mastoidectomy is a lifesaving operation and is not

performed to improve hearing. The surgeon's objective is to remove infected tissue from the middle ear and the mastoid bone. It is often performed on patients with chronic otitis media where the drainage is persistent and has caused a progressive spread of the infection. It usually results in a loss of hearing of approximately 40 to 60 dB at all frequencies in the speech spectrum.

STAPES SURGERY

"Stapes mobilization" involves freeing the stapes from a fixed position in the cochlea. The surgery is performed through the external canal and into the middle ear with the help of a powerful microscope. The eardrum is surgically removed but replaced following the operation. The success rate is reportedly high at first (85 to 90 percent), but declines in time. In many cases, the stapes is again fixated.[105-107]

"Stapedectomy" involves removal of all or a portion of the stapes (the footplate) that is connected to the cochlea (at the oval window). A graft is then placed over the oval window that leads into the cochlea and the contained fluid. A wire is then inserted from the graft to the incus.

Stapedectomy surgery appears to have a far more lasting effect than stapes mobilization, according to many surgeons. It generally takes six months to reveal if such surgery has been successful. However, we must bear in mind that this has been developed only in the past 20 years and the true long-lasting effects may not be known for some time.

The operation is considered to be successful if the patient has increased hearing acuity, increased (or at least not decreased) speech discrimination and no complications as a result of the surgery. However, postoperative dizziness, vertigo, imbalance, faint tinnitus, and fullness in the ear may occur in even the most successful surgical treatment.

FENESTRATION

The fenestration operation was developed in the 1930's to compensate for a conductive problem with the stapes. As a result of otosclerosis, the stapes footplate (that is, the part that enters the cochlea) becomes locked and unable to move enough to transmit sound properly to the cochlea.

It was believed that if another section of the vestibule (of which the cochlea is part) contained a window (called a fenestra) much like the one where the stapes footplate enters the cochlea, bypassing the stapes altogether could allow sound to enter through the new window. This led to making a window in one of the three semicircular canals (responsible for our balance).

The surgical procedure involves removing the bone in the middle ear area to expose a part of the horizontal semicircular canal. A tiny window surgically created in the horizontal canal is then covered with a skin graft taken from the external ear canal. Hence, sound no longer travels from the eardrum to the malleus to the incus to the stapes and into the inner ear. Sound now can travel directly to the new window of the semicircular canal and be directed into the cochlea, bypassing the former middle ear sound system completely.

The hazards of this procedure include the risk of total loss of hearing. The length of hospital stay is usually between five and seven days. If the operation is successful hearing should be improved immediately with recognizable improvement over a period of a few weeks. Since the operation centers around the semicircular canals, dizziness often follows the procedure. Within a period of about three months, though, the ear usually heals completely. However, due to the cavity that is created by fenestration, it is important to have the ear cleaned out about twice a year to prevent infection.

The failure of a fenestration generally occurs within a year as a result of closure of the window, thereby preventing sound from entering the inner ear.

The operation is not difficult in the hands of a skilled surgeon, but it is no longer the preferred method of handling otosclerosis or other conductive impairments. The stapes surgery has been more effective and presently is the preferred method. One of the drawbacks to fenestration is that regardless of the success of the operation, the patient always is left with at least a 21 to 30 dB hearing loss, whereas with stapes surgery, hearing can return to within normal limits. If the fenestration is able to hold for one year, the prognosis for its continued success is very good.

OTOSCLEROSIS

Otosclerosis is a disease of the bony structure surrounding the cochlea. There may or may not be associated conductive hearing loss with the disease. In many postmortem observations of the inner ear, otosclerosis was noted but no prior history of hearing impairment had ever been recorded when the patients had been alive. However, in diagnosed cases of clinical otosclerosis, as much as 50 to 60 dB of hearing loss may exist. Otosclerosis most often affects the lower frequencies first, but eventually may affect all the major frequencies within the speech spectrum.

Otosclerosis is usually first noticed about the age of 18 and is rare in children under 10. It occurs most frequently in people between the ages of 39 and 49, with an incidence much higher among white women than white men (and reportedly in no more than one percent of black men and women) in the United States. One census reveals that the incidence of otosclerosis was nearly double in the 1960's as compared to the previous decade, but no certain explanation has been offered.

In about 50 percent of the cases, otosclerosis is reportedly hereditary. However, the cause of the disease is unknown. It can be progressive and often takes a number of years to become noticeable. The hearing loss is always initially conductive in type but recent evidence indicates that otosclerosis also produces sensorineural hearing impairment since the cochlea is directly affected. Tinnitus is often a very bothersome condition of the disease. The most common procedure for surgical repair of otosclerosis is stapes surgery.[108,109]

MENIERE'S DISORDER

Meniere's Disorder* is a loss of hearing most often in one ear. It affects men between the ages of 40 and 60 more often than women. Meniere's is of the sensorineural type and is

*Recently, the American Medical Association has stated that Meniere's is a syndrome or disorder and is more accurately described and referred to as such rather than referring to the condition as Meniere's Disease, since it is not a disease.

possibly the result of an imbalance in fluid pressure in the inner ear. The hearing loss in Meniere's Disorder is intermittent. Hearing may fluctuate—some days hearing is good, other days it is poor. The loss may appear at all of the frequencies throughout the speech spectrum with the greatest amount of loss in the lower frequencies. The hearing loss may eventually become permanent. There are attacks of vertigo, nausea, fullness of the ears, and disturbing tinnitus described as the roar of an ocean. Recruitment, an abnormally rapid increase in the sensation of sound, may also occur. Due to the high degree of distortion that recruitment produces and the fluctuating nature of the hearing loss, a hearing aid does not always control the hearing problem adequately.

Nervous tension is one of the most frequent symptoms in Meniere's Disorder, and it has been suggested that attacks are less likely to occur if the victim remains quiet and relaxed.

Although there are some surgical procedures available with qualified success, there appears to be no treatment for Meniere's Disorder itself. That is, there is no "cure-all" treatment recognized as "the treatment" for Meniere's Disorder. Many specialists prescribe medication to control the vertigo or nausea. Intravenous injections of the vitamin B complex are also sometimes given. The balance mechanism (the labyrinth) in the inner ear has been surgically destroyed in cases when vertigo or tinnitus has been so debilitating that the victim is in constant agony. Total loss of hearing occurs in such labyrinthine destruction. Unfortunately, not all such surgery has proven effective in eliminating the tinnitus or vertigo. Once performed, the procedure is irreversible[110,111] (see case history ten, p. 153).

Recently, more effective surgical procedures have been used with greater success. The labyrinth is not destroyed, and the hearing can be stabilized and sometimes improved.

Chapter V
HEARING AIDS

PART I: MYTH OR FACT?

The first symptoms of difficulty most often encountered by hard of hearing people are the need for television or radio levels at greater intensities, general strain to hear, accusations that voices are too soft, frequent requests for repeats, a tendency to favor the better ear (if one is better) or cupping the hand around an ear (which actually does increase intensity).

Another very frequent indication of hearing loss is the inability to tell where a sound is coming from. This difficulty includes such sounds as the bark of a dog, the call of a friend from a distance, a knock on a door, etc. There have even been automobile accidents resulting from a driver's inability to determine from which direction a siren was approaching. Auto accidents have also resulted from a driver's inability to hear an emergency vehicle siren until it was too late. Sirens and many other sounds in our environment are high-pitched. If a high frequency loss exists, the possibility of not hearing sirens or other high frequency sounds is quite likely. As with any hearing loss, the eyes must compensate for what the ears miss.

There is no known medical cure or treatment for the type of sensorineural hearing loss produced by long-term noise exposure. The loss simply is ever-present and may necessitate more careful attention to the particulars of conversation.

Knowing the topic of conversation and observing the speaker's lips for visual cues will make hearing and understanding easier. The body also speaks with gestures and facial expressions (and general body movements), so these should be observed for meaning.

There should be absolutely no "bluffing" when it comes to hearing. There should be no hesitation to ask people to repeat and no embarrassment if it is necessary. People should be informed of an existing hearing problem—it should not be concealed. Hiding the loss only encourages the expectation that what is spoken will be heard and understood. Such a fallacy can only end up fooling the person hiding the loss. Continued bluffing is not possible. Once others are aware of a hearing difficulty, they can speak more slowly, more distinctly and with greater intensity.

REALIZING THE LOSS

Motivation is a basic factor that must underlie resolving the emotions involved with a hearing problem. Carl Jung, a Swiss psychiatrist, once told a patient who was suffering from a condition of chronic alcoholism that he could not help him until he was ready to help himself. That meant reaching a level that was so nonobstructive, so unopposing, so undenying as to be receptive to assistance. It took this patient two years without therapy, all alone, with nights so drunk they were forgotten, before he returned to Jung begging for more help or a cure. Jung inspired the alcoholic to start what is now Alcoholics Anonymous (AA).

Similarly, when dealing with a problem stemming from a hearing loss, there must be a basic need from within to seek help. A good friend can't help. A mother can't help. No one can until an individual has reached the crossroads of cooperation, desire and receptivity to help.

THE HEARING AID

Aside from specific training in listening (auditory training), speech (lip) reading or aural rehabilitation, the only proven, qualified non-medical treatment for sensorineural hearing impairment is a hearing aid.

As explained earlier, there is treatment for conductive hearing loss in about 90 percent of the cases and most people prefer surgery over wearing an aid. Nonetheless, there are people who do have conductive hearing impairments who prefer a hearing aid rather than taking the small risks of surgery. Also, if surgery is not successful, the only alternative is a hearing aid. People with a conductive loss usually respond quite favorably to amplification because their ability to understand speech is not impaired. Therefore, if sounds are made loud enough, they will not have difficulty understanding them.

The 1976 total sales of hearing instruments in the United States was approximately 600,000. Sales have been on the increase annually. Although more people are seeking help of this kind each year, more than ten times as many people could benefit from amplification, yet they do not seek help. The average person affected by hearing loss waits five years before reaching that "basic level" that Jung describes as fundamental. Research has revealed that amplification for a hearing loss is associated with better adjustment to the hearing difficulty. Therefore, amplification should be strongly considered when it is indicated.

PSYCHOSOCIAL EFFECTS
OF WEARING A HEARING AID

Somehow, there is an irony in the fact that Americans are far more receptive to wearing eyeglasses at any age than wearing hearing aids. There should be no more vanity in wearing one than the other. Strangely enough, glasses have become so widely used (and accepted) that to many they are considered a mark of distinction. However, in the minds of many potential users, a hearing aid is often equated with a wheelchair. There are two important reasons why: 1) a person's self-consciousness about the instrument (psychological effect) and 2) other people's awareness of the instrument (sociological effect). It is interesting to observe people who speak louder when they see a hard of hearing person with an aid. It should not be necessary since the purpose of the aid is to offer amplification without increased vocal strain by others. Speaking louder will often distort the voice and actually produce an effect opposite of making one's voice more distinguishable, particularly when this signal is carried through a mechanical device.

NATURAL QUALITY SOUND AND PRECISION INSTRUMENTS

Many manufacturers of hearing instruments produce high quality products that have helped millions of people. Even so, care should be taken by the purchaser not to maintain unrealistic expectations about the benefit that is available from amplification. Oftentimes, the user expects to hear as he used to hear. Disappointment is often inevitable in persons with such expectations. A hearing aid may be able to bring impaired hearing back to within normal limits, but the quality of sound may not be quite what it used to be nor what was anticipated.

The vast majority of people with impaired hearing suffer from a high frequency hearing problem (making consonant sounds difficult to hear). Since the very nature of this impairment is one of quality ("I can hear but I don't understand"), the objective is to provide some significant degree of restoration of quality. This requires amplification of just those frequencies that are impaired without amplifying other frequencies that don't need it. The fitting requires precision, because distortion or tolerance problems may result when a hearing aid produces amplification at frequencies where hearing is normal. Depending on the extent of impairment in the high frequencies, a hearing aid may or may not be of benefit.

It is very unlikely that any hearing aid currently on the market could benefit a high frequency sensorineural hearing loss that begins at 2000 Hz or higher. If the hearing loss commences around 1500 Hz, there is a good possibility of help from a hearing aid properly fitted, but not all candidates benefit. If the impairment begins at frequencies of 1000 Hz or lower, most people can look forward to satisfaction from amplification. Benefit from a hearing aid, particularly with high frequency impairment, depends upon the product, the internal specifications of the aid, the ability of the person fitting the aid and ultimately the attitude of the user towards accepting the whole idea of benefit from a prosthetic device (which will require patience and cooperation on the user's part to give it all a chance to work).

THE HEARING AID MARKET

Unfortunately, over the years, hearing aid dealers have been strongly criticized for their high-priced products and services, as well as for taking advantage of consumers. The criticism seems to have been generalized to *all* dealers, and this simply is not the case. Many dealers in business for several years in large cities around the United States are competent. Although there are almost no mandatory educational courses required to become a hearing aid dealer, most dispensers in business for some time have learned their trade through experience rather than any formal training.

As in any business, there are some companies that are more interested in gross volume of sales than individual service. This group within the hearing aid industry has unfortunately led to a great deal of suspicion of the entire industry and some loss of faith. The companies responsible for incurring the overwhelming bulk of abuses are those that promote door-to-door solicitation. In fact, such companies rank on top in the hearing aid industry in terms of gross sales and profits, but understandably suffer from the worst reputation by the public and other dealers as well. A few of these national companies have been responsible for creating a false image of hearing aid dealers as a whole because they have so many brand-name retail branches in major cities in the United States. Part II of this chapter discusses these particular types of companies.

The trend and future of the hearing aid industry is a strongly controversial point. More and more of the present 6,000 hearing aid offices (comprising 15,000 people) are closing their doors to business each year. The average age of the dealer is 55 and there are extremely few young people taking over or coming into this industry. At the same time, there have been far more audiologists trained at the post-graduate college level than there is employment for. Even so, the less than 5,000 audiologists cannot meet the demand for aids plus service that present hearing aid dealers are handling.

The United States government is currently involved in

legislation that would require a consumer of hearing aids to be evaluated by an audiologist prior to the purchase of the aid. Such laws, if enacted and enforced, would provide greater protection for the individuals purchasing the aids. These laws would be no threat to the majority of hearing aid dealers and would essentially eliminate the unethical practices of door-to-door solicitation of hearing aids (see Appendix I).

AUDIOLOGISTS AND PHYSICIANS

Physicians are doctors trained in the practice of medicine and/or surgery. They do not have training in the complex methods and procedures used in clinical audiology. They also have no formal training whatsoever in regard to hearing aids. When a well-meaning physician refers a patient directly to a hearing aid dealer, he bypasses the professional services offered by an audiologist. In such cases, the physician is depriving his patient of better care, leading to additional abuses that hearing aid users might be subjected to.

PART II: THE PURCHASE

More than 90 percent of all hearing aid users are people with sensorineural hearing impairments.[112,113] This group accounts for more than two hundred and fifty million dollars poured into the purchase of hearing aids and related services in the United States annually.[114] One brand-name hearing aid company, one of the largest in the United States, has retail stores that gross more than a quarter of a million dollars annually. This company, and others like it, have "field men" who solicit business from "leads" that are given to them by recent purchasers. They could have your name! Another successful technique for gathering leads is through ads that appear in local newspapers with cut-out postal paid response cards that might read something like: "THE TERRIFIC-EAR . . . a new hearing aid with microcircuitry will give you natural hearing again. No cords. No tubes. No wires. If you would like more information on this brand new, highly scientifically designed instrument, please fill out the attached card. . . ."

Many weeks may pass and you may have just about forgotten that you requested information when, without warning, there will be a man at your door claiming to be following up on your request for information on the TERRIFIC-EAR. You may insist that the card stated there would be literature sent, not a salesman. He may try to let you forget it by promising you a free hearing test to see if you might possibly need a hearing aid. The salesman at this point (and the company he represents) is *guilty of false and misleading advertising* if no literature was in fact mailed. You will almost certainly find yourself a victim of this "gentleman." He may refer to himself as an audiologist. If he does, that is illegal (misrepresentation).

ENCOUNTER WITH A SALESMAN

One anonymous clinical audiologist filled out the type of previously described card he found in a local newspaper and mailed it expecting literature to appear in the mail. It didn't. He was contacted by a salesman via a phone call one evening, about a month and a half after his request. The company was liable for false and misleading advertising because no literature was received. This company had already been taken to court on several counts of misrepresentation. The audiologist decided to feign a hearing loss that would, by the mere high frequency nature, be too far above the critical speech frequencies to be benefitted by amplification. In addition, such a hearing loss is often not detectable by the afflicted individual and poses no real problem. The salesman on the phone inquired to his interest in the TERRIFIC-EAR. The audiologist reported that he was told upon release from the army that he had a high frequency hearing loss in both ears as a result of exposure to tanks (when actually the audiologist had normal hearing and no such exposure). The salesman asked what his livelihood was and he stated that he was an artist (when in fact he was a nationally certified, professionally employed, clinical audiologist). The salesman on the phone stated that the hearing loss sounded like "perceptual deafness" and that he would set up a time for their "hearing aid audiologist" (now an illegal title for a hearing aid salesman) to come over and give a free hearing test. It was refused by the audiologist but the salesman was persistent. The audiologist stated that he expected literature, not a phone call. The salesman ignored his comment and insisted that the hearing test would not cost a dime, nor would there by any "high pressure sales" whatsoever. With such sincerity and reassurance, the audiologist complied.

A date was agreed upon for the salesman to come over to the audiologist's home. A tape recorder was hidden in the living room with two hidden microphones to catch the salesman's voice from wherever he might be standing. In addition, a third party was present as witness to the events. At precisely seven-thirty, a salesman arrived with a gentle knock.

The following are only excerpts of relevant conversation that are intended as serious warnings against such purchases in the home, particularly hearing aids bought on a nonmedical referral. I have altered the company name in the following section in order to protect myself from challenging litigation and in the process, unfortunately, have provided a little shelter for the guilty. As you read, bear in mind that 60 percent of all hearing aid sales are made in the home in a fashion similar to the following kind of solicitation:[115]

Salesman: Hi! I'm Mr. Davis from the Belberg Hearing Aid Company. May I come in?

For appearance, Mr. Davis is best described as looking like "Columbo" in a new tie. He was carrying a portable audiometer (machine to test hearing), was on the plump side, the short side, and probably the not-too-bright side. After testing the audiologist's hearing:

Mr. Davis: Gee. I hate to tell you this, but you have one heck of a loss.

Audiologist: Oh come on! I hear okay. It never really bothers me. Only when I'm around a lot of noise, like at a rock and roll concert. Then I can't hear. You know?

Mr. Davis: No. I know what I see here. You don't hear well in other
               places either.
Audiologist: I don't?
Mr. Davis: That's right. Now is the time to do something about it or
               you will soon develop a serious hearing loss, much worse
               than it is already.

Mr. Davis has made a medical evaluation that he has no
legal right to make. His comment is not only untrue—it is
illegal. A decision *not* to buy a hearing aid has no bearing on
whether or not one's hearing gets better or worse.

Audiologist: Do you think I ought to at least see my doctor or maybe
               go to one of the hearing clinics and have my ears
               checked out there?
Mr. Davis: (Vulgarity omitted) . . . Don't be ridiculous! Absolutely
               not! They will give you the exact same test I did and they
               will charge you more than fifty dollars while mine is
               free.

A sound treated room is necessary to reveal the baseline
hearing threshold of a person. It cannot be conducted in an
environment that is noisy or on a machine that is out of
calibration. Also, hearing tests may be free, performed at local
speech and hearing university-connected centers. They are
often approximately fifteen dollars in a doctor's office carried
out by an audiologist in a soundproof room. Mr. Davis has
provided false and misleading information.

Audiologist: Well, do you think I ought to go to the Veterans
               Administration Hospital at least to see about the hearing
               loss? I was in Nam and being a veteran I would think I
               could get some help there.
Mr. Davis: My good friend, I wouldn't steer you wrong. They most
               likely won't be able to help you. Let me ask if you were
               discharged in perfect health?
Audiologist: No. I was shot in the leg.
Mr. Davis: Are you collecting compensation for it now?
Audiologist: No.
Mr. Davis: Did you put in a claim for a hearing loss?

Audiologist: No, because it wasn't until recently that my ringing started to get worse which made me wonder about my hearing.

Mr. Davis: That's it then. Won't do you any good now to go to the V.A., but of course you can try. Their hearing aids cost four hundred dollars and besides, it's probably too late to do anything about it.

Mr. Davis has borderlined a federal offense. Again, he has provided misinformation. All veterans are entitled to a complete audiological workup at a V.A. outpatient clinic or hospital facility equipped for such evaluations. This is done at no personal expense whatsoever to the veteran. The government picks up the tab to cover travel costs to and from the facility (by car, train, plane or whatever), as well as room and board if necessary in the city where the evaluation is done. Veterans found to have a service-connected hearing impairment are eligible for a free hearing aid and lifetime follow-up as well as any necessary medical and rehabilitative assistance. Under no circumstances does the V.A. sell hearing aids, which Mr. Davis implied. Also, it is never too late to put a claim in for compensation due to defective hearing caused during time in the service.

Mr. Davis: This hearing aid here will also prevent your hearing from getting worse.

Audiologist: You mean if I don't buy a hearing aid, my hearing may get worse because of not buying one?

Mr. Davis: That's correct. The aid stimulates your membranes inside the ear. Way inside. Can even make you less likely to get the flu.

Composure was difficult for the audiologist. Hearing research reveals no scientific data to support the hypothesis that a hearing aid stimulates hair cells and nerve endings to a point of "preventing" further deterioration. The statement that an aid can prevent the flu or any other condition is absolutely preposterous. It is incorrect and unfounded. On the contrary, an improperly fitted hearing instrument can actually cause further hearing loss, particularly in young infants who cannot regulate the volume. Over-amplification in any way, whether through a hearing aid to a damaged ear or through the air to a normal ear, can have grave effects upon hearing.

Mr. Davis proceeded to place a hearing aid into the audiologist's ear. The hearing aid had an extremely high internal noise level that was apparent at once to the audiologist, but could be easily passed off by a smooth salesman as "nothing unusual." The noise from the instrument sounded like a muffled, distant, roaring windstorm. Mr. Davis utilized the art of suggestion to the point of near-nausea. The third party witnessing the events (also revealed later on the playback tape) reported that Mr. Davis increased the intensity of his voice as soon as the aid was in the ear. His speech was also unusually more distinct!

Audiologist: I hear a hum somewhere. Or wind.

Mr. Davis: Now. Look at that. See? For the first time in I'll bet years you're going to hear all the things you've been missing. You're probably hearing the wind through the porch door here. See? You have to get used to a hearing aid. It's . . .

Audiologist: (Closing the porch door tightly.) No! I still hear it. It's in the aid.

Mr. Davis: Oh, wait a minute, you're hearing the refrigerator motor. I find that most of my patients discover this when they first put on a hearing aid. But you have to get used . . .

Audiologist: Used to it? (Opening refrigerator door and turning dial to "defrost.") I still hear the . . . noise! What are you trying to sell me?

Mr. Davis: I want you to know I have two degrees and am trained to know what I'm talking about. I have an A.D. degree for one . . .

Mr. Davis revealed his state license to dispense hearing aids. He stated that it was his first degree. He never explained what the other degree was. A license to dispense hearing aids is not a degree. Also, using the descriptive term "patients"

91

suggests a medical association for which Mr. Davis could have none to permit such an inference. Mr. Davis is a salesman, not a physician nor paramedical professional.

Realizing he was slowly losing a sale, Mr. Davis dropped the price of the "demonstrator model" from three hundred to one hundred and twenty dollars. When that didn't work, he offered a three-day trial period with a deposit of "only" fifty dollars. The salesman was escorted to the door where he exited on his own accord. Mr. Davis never did demonstrate the TERRIFIC-EAR. He used a bait and switch technique in sales which is illegal—coming on with an inexpensive item and switching to a more expensive one. Within a matter of sixty minutes, Mr. Davis became liable on one count of bait and switch, one count of misleading advertising, three counts of false claims and four counts of misrepresentation.

THE FOLLOW-UP

Follow-up letters are a standard procedure in "no-sale" solicitation as previously described. However, the audiologist received only one letter that was not very sales oriented. No further correspondence was received. It was later strongly suspected that Mr. Davis discovered that he had been to the home of an audiologist and discontinued any further correspondence. Usually customers are pestered by mail from such companies. It also is standard practice for salesmen to return to the door within a year.

The real culprit is the company for which Mr. Davis works. They encourage and promote this kind of selling and often set up sales quotas for salesmen to meet each month.

OFFENSES

Every company that promotes home solicitation has been charged and penalized by the Federal Trade Commission (FTC). It should be pointed out that exceptionally few hearing aid manufacturers encourage such selling practices, but the few that do engage in this type of approach to the consumer have been charged with offenses that include: false claims, misleading advertising, misrepresentation, exclusive dealing, coercion in contracts, bait and switch, intimidation of dealers and restraint of trade. A few bad apples may well be found in almost any bushel. But when the few bad apples cause the entire bushel to be suspect, it is imperative that the bad apples be sorted out and looked at more carefully.

NO LICENSE TO DISPENSE

One of the major reasons so many home solicitation abuses have occurred within the hearing aid industry is that legislation protecting the consumer from home solicitation either does not exist or is poorly enforced. As late as 1976, ten states still had so few regulations that any man, regardless of educational background or training, could open an office and sell hearing aids without a license. He could test hearing and sell aids to anyone he felt needed one, at any price he felt he could get.

THE 65+ YEAR-OLD VICTIM

An investigation by the Retired Professional Action Group (RPAG), sponsored by Ralph Nader, revealed that 50 percent of all aids in the United States are purchased by people age 65 or older.[116] In 1971, this group had average individual incomes of less than twenty-two hundred dollars yearly. Considering that the price of many aids bought from salesmen in the home is five-hundred to one-thousand dollars each, the elderly are an unfortunately vulnerable target for any door-to-door solicitor looking for his bonanza. There are more than 21 million Americans over the age of 65, two million of whom live in rest homes of which 90 percent suffer from significant hearing impairments[117] (see Appendix IV).

CONSUMER PROTECTION

As discussed in Part I of this chapter, we are rapidly approaching a time when each state will require everyone to be examined by an audiologist before purchasing a hearing aid. Such legislation would then force the largest violators (the home solicitors) to cease present methods of selling. Sale of a hearing aid through the mail would also then be illegal. Presently, 70 percent of the consumers who buy aids do so without the advice or consultation of either an audiologist or physician. The Department of Health, Education and Welfare (HEW) has estimated that the cost of hearing loss in the United States runs more than four hundred ten million dollars annually for the education, management and compensation of all hearing impaired individuals. By 1980, this could reach over half a billion dollars annually.[118]

The National Bureau of Standards has estimated that the list price of an average aid is three hundred fifty dollars. Of the approximate 600,000 hearing aids sold in 1976, if the price were actually three hundred fifty dollars (a conservative figure), then two hundred ten million dollars were spent on aids alone. That is more than 50 percent of the HEW's estimated four hundred ten million dollars spent annually in the total care of the hearing impaired.

MAIL-ORDER HEARING AIDS

Mail-order hearing aid purchases are as bad an idea as a purchase in the home. RPAG reported that the average customer visits the hearing aid office seven times before achieving satisfaction from a hearing aid. Although this may be a rather high estimate of visits, when a hearing instrument is bought through the mail, service on the unit may be absolutely impossible or grossly inadequate if available at all. Personal service is unequivocally necessary for the purchase and maintenance of a hearing aid. A very simple problem may result in an unnecessarily large expense if the aid is sent back to the mail-order company. Hearing aids that are advertised for forty-nine dollars and fifty cents or sixty-nine dollars and fifty cents made in Japan are as unwise a purchase as eyeglasses that used to be marketed through similar ads many years ago offering inexpensive correction of vision for near- or far-sighted people. Just as optometrists have been instrumental in the fitting of eyeglasses, seeking out trained individuals in the fitting of hearing aids is important.

IDENTICAL AIDS NOT IDENTICAL

The internal specifications for the same make and model hearing aid can vary so greatly that for all intents and purposes they could be two entirely different instruments from two different manufacturers. Present laws permit such variation of the same make and model. RPAG reported that the Veterans Administration finds seven out of every one hundred hearing aids don't work at all, not to mention the permissible variations within the same make and model. The V.A. receives and fits about 7,000 hearing aids each year. Hence, nearly 500 brand new aids are returned each year to various manufacturers because they do not work at all. And the V.A. reportedly uses the best aids available. This can only let the imagination run wild with thoughts of what door-to-door salesmen might be working with, not having the control over aids nor the restrictions that the V.A. method of dispensing imposes.

WHAT IS IN AN AID WORTH $350?

The actual components of a hearing aid consist of a microphone, a magnetic receiver, about three transistors, some seven resistors, about six capacitors, less than three cents' worth of wire and a plastic shell to hide it all in. The total cost of parts is about twenty-five dollars. Labor, advertising and distribution of the average hearing aid would bring the price to about fifty dollars. The aid is then sold by a manufacturer to a retail store at approximately one hundred dollars. The retailer then sells the product to the public for more than a 200 percent markup.[119]

GREATER PRICE EQUALS GREATER QUALITY?

The reason that hearing aids are so expensive is because so few of them are sold by the many hearing aid dispensers throughout the country. An estimated 6,000 dealers selling 600,000 hearing aids at, let's say, three hundred fifty dollars each is approximately thirty-five thousand dollars per hearing aid office, gross earnings, out of which at least one, and generally two (or more) other people have to be paid. So the prices remain high for apparently justifiable reasons.

Nonetheless, quality cannot be equated with price in hearing aids. The same instrument may sell for 10 different prices in the same city. There is a manufacturer's suggested retail price, but few have a maximum price set. There is the story of a man showing off his brand-new hearing aid to a friend. The owner of the instrument was bragging about how much it had cost him: "The most expensive one on the market," he claimed. "What kind is it?" his friend inquired. "It's about three-thirty," the proud owner answered.

THE SIZE

Recent technological advances indicate some promising results for all-in-the-ear models. However, the overwhelming majority of such aids at this time generally have a higher degree of distortion than behind-the-ear types and a reduced amount of power in addition to a poorer quality of sound. In smaller aids, fewer transistors, resistors and capacitors are able to be squeezed into the tiny plastic shell. A lack of enough of these components contributes to significant low frequency distortion. An unpublished V.A. study in Los Angeles reported that all-in-the-ear aids comprised 4 percent of the total aids dispensed in 1970 (as compared to 71 percent of other ear-level instruments).

The physical size of the hearing aid varies depending upon the type that is selected. All-in-the-ear aids are the smallest aids available and are generally no larger than the tip of your index finger. Although they are the smallest aids, they are not necessarily the least visible. Behind-the-ear aids can be hidden completely behind the ear with very low visibility (only the tube and the earmold are visible), and are usually no longer than two inches.

Eyeglass hearing aids are not my preference for amplification for the reasons given in the answer to Question 30 (see chapter six). However, the primary benefit of this aid is complete invisibility of its components, which are constructed within the stem of the glasses.

The largest hearing aid, and the type that most people associate with a hearing loss, is the body aid. It is approximately the size of one or two packs of cigarettes. A wire transmits the sound from the aid to the ear. This type of aid offers the greatest amount of amplification, and is used primarily in cases of profound hearing loss.

TOLERANCE PROBLEMS

More than 85 percent of the hearing aids sold in the United States are ear-level instruments.[120] Most people are overfitted with hearing aids. Like automobiles, aids come with different amounts of power already built in. The amount of power can be regulated by a volume wheel. However, when the power is extremely limited, as when driving a small car with a small engine up a steep incline, it doesn't matter how hard or long the gas pedal is to the floor (or the volume wheel is at full power). Only so much power can be tapped, predetermined by the size of the driving unit. Few people are underfitted with aids in this way. Many people are fitted with hearing aids that are equivalent to a large luxury car, with more power available than will ever be utilized.

Most new users have a tendency to keep the volume of an aid lower than what is actually indicated for maximum benefit. Since nearly all ears with sensorineural hearing impairments suffer from recruitment (a condition marked by an abnormal increase in the intensity of sounds), this is one factor in adjusting to an aid. But this is generally coupled with an even more significant factor—too many aids are fitted with too much power. These two factors determine the degree of difficulty in adjusting to and tolerating an aid. A 1967 survey revealed that 58 percent of former hearing aid users had stopped wearing their aids altogether for reasons of discomfort (due to the high internal power of the aid).[121]

THE TRIAL AND PURCHASE

When a hearing aid is indicated, it should be taken out on a trial basis for a rental fee (usually one dollar per day per aid) for at least 30 days. The initial investment is then only thirty dollars which is applied to the purchase price of the instrument at the end of the trial, or forfeited if the aid is not purchased. The trial period establishes whether or not an aid can help compensate for the hearing loss and determines which particular instrument is likely to provide the maximum benefit.

The recommendation for a hearing aid should originate

from an audiologist, employed in most large university or community speech and hearing clinics as well as in ear, nose and throat hospital clinics. Many are also in private practice in major cities throughout the United States. If an audiologist cannot be contacted, a speech and hearing center would have information on who to see. For protection of the consumer, it is *not* a good idea to walk into a hearing aid office as though it were a department store and shop without knowledge of whether or not a hearing aid can fundamentally even be of benefit.

Chapter VI
ANSWERS TO YOUR QUESTIONS

As a practicing clinical audiologist I have been confronted with a wide array of questions about hearing problems. In this chapter, I present those questions that I feel are the most important and the most frequently asked, and I have answered them in greater detail than a clinical setting would allow.

QUESTIONS ABOUT HEARING AND HEARING PROBLEMS

#1   **Q:** *My husband always talks so loud, even in ordinary conversation, that when we're in public, it's embarrassing to friends we're with. I'm used to it after all these years. But an audiologist saw him and said that it was because he had a hearing loss. He won't get a hearing aid. How can I quiet his unrestrained volume?*

A: You can't. Speech and hearing are as inseparable as the startled response from a pin that sticks you. The reactions to both are reflexive, automatic—not in the conscious control of the person responding. Your husband no doubt speaks in a seemingly boisterous manner because of his inability to *monitor* his own vocal intensity. His voice may not appear unusually loud to him because his hearing loss prevents him from hearing himself well. As a result, his voice increases in intensity. If he spoke at a level that the normal hearing person would want him to, he might feel as though he were speaking far too softly. A hearing aid, properly fitted, could very successfully bring the volume of his voice back down to within conversational limits. It is not uncommon for such a person to be treated for vocal strain, abuse, nodules, sore throats and other laryngeal problems stemming from a hearing loss.

There is also equipment available to provide an individual with information on vocal intensity. Some biofeedback machines and the "Florida I" provide visual representation of excessive volume.

#2   **Q:** *I have a long-standing hearing loss that has gotten worse over the years. It was caused, I presume, from 25 years of exposure to loud noises around a gas station I own and work in. I don't wear a hearing aid. I tried one a few years ago but sounds were so loud I couldn't stand it. I can't hear and understand people because either their voices aren't clear enough or my ear hurts if they speak up too loud. What's wrong?*

A: It appears that you have a high frequency hearing loss, but of course an audiological evaluation would be necessary to determine that. Noise exposure, though, is most often the destroyer of high frequencies. If you presumably hear all right in the lower frequencies, sound needn't be louder than normal to be heard in this range. But sound in the higher frequencies will have to be louder to be perceived. These sounds are in the range of consonants, but as a person speaks to you, it obviously is not possible to make the consonants louder while not altering the acoustics of the vowels. While a hearing aid may improve your hearing by making sounds louder, the human voice becomes distorted when greatly raised. When people try to increase their voices, thinking you will hear better, what they're actually doing may be the opposite. An abnormal increase in the voice makes understanding of speech more difficult. Your ear wants *certain* sounds louder without increased intensity in other sounds, and it can't get it without a hearing aid—and even this may not resolve the problem for you.

Other than trying a hearing aid successfully used by many

of my patients with the kind of problem you describe, speech-reading and aural rehabilitation (how to listen) are your basic alternatives.

#3 **Q:** *My wife complains that I turn the television up too loud. It doesn't seem that loud to me but even the neighbors have mentioned it. What can I do?*

A: Assuming that you do not have a hearing aid to amplify television, there are ways to resolve not being able to hear the television at the same time eliminating family conflict that often revolves around "volume."

An earphone can be worn that can allow the rest of the family to rest in peace. There is also a rather small speaker that can be used. It is connected to the sound system of the television (or radio), and via a wire, provides enough distance to maintain the speaker next to a chair or sofa. The volume of the television can be adjusted to the particular viewer's liking. On many such units, there is also a tone control. (See Appendix VI for purchasing information.)

#4 **Q:** *I have worked around very loud noises for about two years in a print shop. I am now occasionally getting ringing in my ears but my otologist and audiologist tell me that my hearing is normal. The audiologist recommended ear protection with large earmuffs, but I can't communicate with my fellow workers with them on. In fact, once I was almost killed because they were shouting at me to get out of the way of a compressor that broke open. I'm afraid to wear the ear protection because I can't hear, even for safety's sake, but I'm also afraid I may lose my hearing. What should I do?*

A: Tinnitus (ringing ears) is one of the first signs of potential hearing damage. The fact that you report it as occasional may indicate a temporary problem if a remedy is found, perhaps by removing noise pollutants or installing filters on equipment. I would encourage you to take some immediate action to resolve your present dilemma—there is no job worth losing your hearing over. If you are to remain on the same job as a printer and if you expect to maintain some semblance of normal hearing you will have to utilize ear protection to the fullest. At the same time, if ear protection means the possibility of not hearing warning signals and may be a threat of severe personal injury, certainly living with a hearing disorder is better than dying with excellent hearing! If there are perhaps times when you can wear the protection without the risk of not hearing warning signals, it should be done. Your employer should be informed of the serious conflict you face and it should be his responsibility to resolve the noise problem.

#5   **Q:** *This may sound strange, but I believe that I hear better in the morning. I am around noise, rather loud, during the day at work. It seems that when I come home in the evening, the noise is still in my ears, even if it's absolutely quiet. Is this possible?*

A: If you are around a significant amount of noise during the day, this can shift your hearing threshold to a less sensitive level. Recovery from noise can take normally from a few hours to a few weeks, depending upon the level of noise and exposure time. However, if the noise is a regular part of your life, the recovery time will require more and more time until eventually you will be out of time at which point the less sensitive level may become your new permanent hearing level (and then that level eventually may become less sensitive as noise exposure continues at harmful intensities).

The fact that you believe you hear better in the morning would indicate that there might have been sufficient recovery time from the noise insult. But when you reach the point when you no longer hear better in the mornings than in the evenings, you may have reached a crossroads of permanent loss of hearing. TAKE PROTECTION FROM NOISE EXPOSURE NOW.

#6   **Q:** *Is it possible that at times I don't hear well because I don't feel well?*

A: Yes. Mental and physical health are important factors in hearing well. You may not listen well at times which in turn causes you to not hear well. If your attention span is short, for whatever reason, and your mind is wandering or preoccupied with thoughts, this does not allow for ideal listening conditions.

Not hearing well because you are not listening well is not a hearing problem; it is a listening problem. If you do not listen, you will not hear. When you "listen," you hear with thoughtful attention. If I say something to you and you answer or react appropriately, I would assume that you were listening to me because you responded appropriately as a result of "hearing" me. This might sound redundant, but it isn't. If you walk outdoors in the midst of a thunder and lightning storm and do not "hear" the rumble of thunder, it isn't because you necessarily have a hearing loss. If you do not listen for thunder, you will not hear it. A more common example is being outdoors and all of a sudden "hearing" the traffic in the background, or the chirping of birds or the sound of wind through the trees. In order to hear, you must *perceive* sound.

If you happen to have a hearing loss, it does not impair your ability to listen unless you choose not to listen. However, it does impair your ability to hear regardless of how hard you try to hear. Hearing then, as we know it, occurs at two levels: the ear receives sound through the process of hearing, and the brain provides meaningful interpretation of the sound through listening.

#7   **Q:** *Other people appear to be more bothered by my hearing loss than I am. I've been told by an audiologist to get a hearing aid but I feel I manage quite satisfactorily without one. What should I do about other people?*

A: For many people like yourself, the problem that is fundamentally your own becomes a shared problem when trying to communicate effectively. There is no substitute for hearing. Speechreading is your basic alternative but it offers quite limited possibilities. "Filling in the gaps" for speech sounds not clearly discriminated nor visually perceived is simply not possible to do for any length of time due to so many variables.

As far as other people go, the most I can suggest is to

inform them you have a hearing problem and would appreciate their consideration in helping you to hear better by speaking a little louder and perhaps more distinctly and slowly. However, the responsibility for your own problem will be shifted to those around you. If you saw a man who could walk quite well with the assistance of a cane, but he preferred that you carried him, would you? Should you? If he can walk with a cane, should anyone carry him? The same can be applied to your hearing. Others may feel that the burden of *your* problem has been selfishly thrust into *their* laps. Why should they have to do all those things to help you hear better if you could benefit from a hearing aid, particularly upon an audiologist's recommendation? The question then is not so much what you should do about other people, but what you might do to help yourself. The best resolution may only come with the assistance of a hearing aid (and speechreading).

#8　**Q:** *Why do I feel so depressed ever since I developed a hearing loss?*

A: Depression is a real problem with any handicap. Gaining an insight into the nature of the problem can perhaps provide an explanation for such a reaction. Sounds that the normal hearing individual takes for granted and considers least important are frequently the very sounds that the hard of hearing person misses most. These are the sounds that help us to orient ourselves in our environment. They may be meaningless until they are no longer audible. Such background sounds as a grandfather clock ticking in the living room, wind chimes outside, the lull of traffic or sound of a motor nearby provide a feeling of security. They are audible at a subconscious level. However, somewhat ironically, a person often becomes conscious of such sounds in their absence. It's like walking into the heart of a jungle expecting to hear all the associated sounds but hearing a dead silence. The sensation may well be awesome. A hard of hearing person lives in a world of partial silence; a world separated from the real world by the absence of sound. This detachment is similar to feelings of severance or loss. A frequent human reaction is depression because orientation has been upset.

Research into sensory deprivation in man (and other animals) has revealed astonishing information on how important our environment is in providing all animals with the necessary means of monitoring themselves. We see ourselves relative to our environment. Many experiments have been carried out on normal functioning humans intentionally deprived of environmental contact. Such isolation has been found to be intolerable. Man has shown decreased motor functioning, changes in personality, altered psychological and nervous system functioning and changes in behavior.

For all intents and purposes, there are five senses. Only two of these five are "distance" senses: auditory and visual. The other three are "close" senses: taste, touch and smell. When one of these distance senses becomes impaired, the effect can be devastating. Our link to the environment is through our senses. It provides a reference for our reality. An impairment to our senses alters our state of awareness. A sensory deprivation is certainly reason for depression. However, it is important not to dwell on the hearing loss.

#9 Q: *I have a sensorineural hearing loss. Will it get worse?*

A: It is a fairly safe bet that anyone with either normal hearing or a sensorineural hearing loss will experience some degree of progressive deterioration in hearing, if from nothing other than our noisy environment alone. Precisely how much decreased hearing acuity will occur over the years is not possible to predict. However, some people seem to have a predisposition for hearing loss and may develop more rapid hearing deterioration than others.

#10 Q: *What can I do if I cannot hear the telephone ring unless I'm in the same room as the phone?*

A: There are many ways to get around this problem. The general offices of most telephone companies in the U.S. offer special services to the hard of hearing. If your particular hearing problem is one of a high frequency nature, the bell in the phone can be replaced with another bell that will ring at a different pitch, presumably where your hearing is more acute. If this is not your particular problem, a "gong" or "alarm" is available. This is like a school bell that rings extremely loud. Many people with even severe hearing impairments can utilize these services in conjunction with the use of a hearing aid. For more information, contact a representative at your local telephone business office.

#11 Q: *I have a habit of getting in the shower and letting a single spray from the showerhead go into my ear canal. I enjoy the sensation; at the same time it has kept my ears clean for 30 years. I have never had to go to a doctor for an ear infection or wax removal. Is this a dangerous practice?*

A: A physician once commented that if what goes in does not hurt, and if it comes back out and that doesn't hurt, it probably is not dangerous (although there are exceptions to this). If a person with a perforated eardrum does that, he is likely to end up as an emergency case in an ear, nose and throat clinic! The method you describe is similar to the method used by otologists in the removal of wax from the ear. The intensity of the spray certainly should not be excessive—it could puncture the eardrum.

#12 Q: *I have a conductive hearing loss in both ears. My surgeon told me he cannot operate a third time on either ear (revisions). The audiologist said that I could probably get along by using only one hearing aid in the poorer ear. I do not hear well at all. Rather than getting a hearing aid, I got a second opinion from another surgeon who said he could operate, but there'd be a 10 percent chance of it worsening after the operation. The original surgeon said the same thing and after surgery the first and second time it wasn't worse; it just wasn't better. How can two reputable surgeons with such success in the community have two entirely different opinions?*

A: Probably nobody knows what is inside your ears better than the surgeon who has operated on them. If that surgeon reported that there is nothing further he can do about your hearing, I would certainly respect his opinion. Either your ear is not capable of handling any further surgery or the surgeon feels *he* is not able to perform further surgery without high risks of losing some hearing. The surgeon making an opinion about additional surgery hopefully has gone through your entire medical history to have a basis for his opinion. If you see other surgeons you may find that you come upon even more opposing opinions. You have to be able to decide who is providing you with the most logical rationale and proceed from there.

#13 **Q:** *I was stricken with sudden deafness in one ear. I've been to several specialists and nobody can suggest how or why it happened. However, I have noticed that ever since it happened, I can no longer tell where people are speaking to me from. Why?*

A: Human beings have two ears for a similar reason they have two eyes. It allows for a third dimension. You cannot have three-dimensional vision (depth perception) with one eye. Extend your index fingers in front of your face, about a foot away at eye level. Close one eye and begin to move one finger away from the face keeping it at eye level. Focus your eye on the finger moving away. If you do this properly, you will realize that the finger moving away from the stationary finger actually does not appear to change in its relative size. Repeat the exercise with both eyes open and focused on the finger moving away and you will realize that the finger now appears to be getting smaller as it moves further away. One eye cannot provide depth perception whereas two eyes can. One ear cannot provide the ability to separate a signal (such as speech) from noise (such as traffic). Two ears allow us to pick out a signal from noise (through a figure-ground relationship). They allow us to discriminate between foreground and background sounds.

The time difference between sound reaching the first ear and then the second ear is the factor that determines localization of sound. The ear nearest the sound source receives the sound first and more intensely. Loss in one ear impairs this ability. The problem you describe is not restricted to ears with total loss. A great many people with high frequency hearing impairments suffer from the same difficulties.

#14 Q: *My favorite drink is a vodka and tonic. I was told by an ear specialist that it could be contributing to my progressive hearing loss and tinnitus. How?*

A: Alcohol is an ototoxic drug and a known cause of ringing in the ears. I would therefore consider reducing your intake of any alcohol per your physician's recommendation.

As for the tonic water that you take with your vodka, this can also be lethal to your inner ear. Tonic water contains quinine, a known destructive chemical to the inner ear. So your favorite drink of a vodka and tonic might best be replaced with something else if you do not want to continue taking the chance that both are contributing to your hearing problem. You might switch to another drink for a few weeks, and if possible, something nonalcoholic, and see if there is any change in either your hearing or ringing. You should work with your physician or ear specialist on this matter.

#15 Q: *Is it safe to fly with a head cold?*

A: If you suffer from congestion and are planning to be aboard an airplane, you should consult your physician or ear specialist regarding the safety of flying during this condition. Most often it is considered unsafe because with a cold and accompanying congestion in the head, the cabin air pressure and decompression can force an infection through the eustachian tube and into the middle ear where a host of problems could develop.

#16 Q: *Every time I fly, my ears get plugged up. Can I do anything about this?*

A: Assuming that you have normal hearing or at least no pathological problem with the ears, you might find doing what I do to be quite helpful. Whenever I fly, due to the decompression within the cabin of the plane, I chew gum at takeoff and landing (a point at which the air pressure of the cabin changes the most). Chewing gum keeps the eustachian tube periodically open so that equalization of pressure within the ears occurs. This can help tremendously to keep the ears from plugging up as you describe.

You might have wondered why stewardesses pass out hard candy during landing and takeoff. It may also be out of courtesy, but it is primarily to relieve the pressure that builds up in the ears. Infants too young to chew candy should be given a bottle. If a bottle is not available, drinking something will relieve the pressure within the ears. Should pain follow decompression, a physician should be consulted.

#17   Q: *How can I be sure that I have a hearing loss without consulting a hearing health professional?*

A: If you can honestly tell yourself that any of the following apply to a listening situation for *you*, you may suspect a hearing loss and should consult your physician, ear specialist or audiologist.

a. General strain to hear, realized by having to lean forward or sit on the edge of a chair.

b. Need to have sentences or parts of sentences repeated, either because you are not sure of what was said or didn't hear it.

c. Other people comment about your hearing by saying things like, "You're not concentrating," or you feel you are not concentrating.

d. A preference for sounds to be louder, including television, radio, music, or others complain that you listen to these at levels greater than they prefer.

e. Find it difficult or impossible to hear the sounds of things you know you used to hear sharply, including your watch ticking, falling rain, blowing wind, a telephone ringing, a doorbell, etc.

f. One ear is better than the other.

g. At times need to cup your hand around your ear or turn your head to favor your better ear and realize you can hear better.

h. Easier to hear men than women or children.

i. Difficulty hearing in an environment that is relatively

noisy, such as in restaurants, at parties or in a room with a loud television or other noises.

j. Tend to pay close attention to lips and gestures of a speaker in order to avoid straining.

k. Socialize less because of anticipated difficulty in listening situations that include going to the theater, luncheons, dinners, meetings, etc.—all of which isolates you more than you care to be.

#18   Q: *My daughter has had chronic ear infections for years. She loves to swim but the physician we see has told her not to swim with the infection. Another physician, in the meantime, suggested that she wear earplugs—the kind that are molded to the ears. Is this practical and effective?*

A: There is controversy on this question by physicians, audiologists and hearing aid dispensers alike. From my own experience, having used both, I can tell you that neither standard earplugs nor molded earplugs* are to be considered effective to the degree that they keep water out of the ear canal. If your daughter is going to wade and not splash in the water, either would no doubt be effective. If she is actually going to swim and get her head into the water, neither will keep water entirely out of the ears.

There are naturally many variables that have to be considered here and only you can decide which of the many variables applies to her: how active is she in the water?; how long is she in the water?; how deep does she go while in the water (does she swim underwater)? The amount of her own activity determines whether to get the inexpensive earplugs or the more expensive plugs that are molded to the ear.

Some additional considerations should also be noted. The cost difference is great. Standard rubber earplugs are generally under five dollars while the molded plugs cost from thirty to fifty dollars. However, because one is molded to the ear, it generally fits better (providing that a good impression of the

---

*Molded earplugs are made by most hearing aid dealers. A soft material is poured into the ear, allowed to harden, removed in a matter of minutes and sent away to a laboratory for preparation.

ear is made). Standard rubber plugs, which can be found in most drugstores, usually only come in sizes small, medium or large, if in fact some places even carry various sizes.

There are certain advantages to both kinds of plugs, other than the fit and the cost. Molded plugs have much more mass than rubber ones. This has one advantage and one disadvantage: the larger mass may keep more water out of the ear canal, but if there is any movement of the jaw or lips the ear canal may move, depending on the amount of motion. You can experience this by putting your finger in your ear and moving your jaw up and down and sideways while puckering your lips and alternately smiling. This motion occurs while swimming and can let water slip around the plug. Since there is greater mass with the molded plug, it tends to move more as one unit while the standard rubber plug, being far more flexible and pliable, can move at one end without greatly disturbing the other end, therefore allowing less water to enter the ear canal (if it fits properly).

Perhaps one of the most important considerations of all is the tendency for standard earplugs to fall out more easily than molded ones which lock into the ear more securely. Depending upon the amount of activity in the water then, this may be a determining factor as to which plug to get.

If your daughter has recently undergone ear surgery, or is being treated for an ongoing ear infection, it may be wisest for her to avoid swimming altogether.

#19   Q: *Is an earache a sign of a hearing loss?*

A: An earache *can* be a sign of a hearing loss or indication of a possible hearing disorder, but not always. Frequently, bruising the ear can produce an earache with no accompanying hearing loss. Earaches can also be caused by an irritation from the use of a cotton swab, or blowing the nose too forcefully (thereby causing a problem with the eustachian tube and/or middle ear pressure). An earache can also be produced by an impacted or infected third molar. In this case, you should consult your dentist or oral surgeon. He may then refer you to an ear specialist.

Some people develop problems with their jaw joint, known as the temporal-mandibular joint. Any disarticulation of the joint can produce a referred pain to the ear. If you are having difficulty chewing and experience a pain in the ear, again, consultation with a medical specialist is encouraged.

It is not terribly infrequent to find a patient who experiences pain in the ear as a result of the common cold. Oftentimes with head colds, there is a production of fluid in the middle ears. Frequently, children with an inflammation of the pharynx or tonsils will develop an earache. In any event, it is always wise to seek medical advice.

#20 **Q:** *I'm just curious about something. A friend of mine has a daughter who is stone deaf. She supposedly can read lips quite well but I find that she frequently gets lost when I speak with her and I have to repeat myself. However, I am amazed she can get along as well as she does. Why does she have so much trouble and will she ever be able to understand speech better than she does?*

A: Speechreading (also referred to as lipreading) is the art of comprehending words through interpretation of the visual cues of a speaker. This includes lip, mouth and jaw movements, facial expressions and gestures. Speechreading is not easy. It requires time to become proficient. The ability to speechread is limited, though. This is primarily due to the low visibility of most speech sounds (an estimated 60 percent of sounds in the English language are either greatly obscured or not visible); many sounds are homophenous (that is, many sounds *visually* appear to be identical, but sound different, such as "bit," "mit" and "pit"); normal conversational speech occurs at a rate faster than the eye is capable of observing (that is, approximately 13 speech sounds are produced per second while the eye can only capture 10 at best);[122] many people articulate the same sounds in different ways (for example, /sh/ can be made with the lips either greatly protruded, retracted or any degree in between); and there can be many environmental limitations such as poor light for observing visual cues or if a speaker's back is turned, or visual obstructions such as a pipe in the mouth or a large mustache hanging over the lip.

Many speechreading teachers have found that the art takes about three years to learn and that progress beyond this point is usually quite slow. If the deaf child you refer to has been speechreading for many years and has had continued instruction in it for many years, she may have reached her plateau whereby there may not be an increase in her ease of speechreading. It is not just deaf and hard of hearing people who utilize speechreading. Even the normal hearing individual is unconsciously reading lips and picking up meaningful visual cues, particularly in noisy environments where auditory input is greatly reduced.

Speechreading ability has been positively correlated with intelligence and general reading ability. A sex difference has also been strongly suggested by many studies indicating that women find it easier to speechread than men.

#21 Q: *My husband and I have normal hearing. Our girl has normal hearing but our boy has a hearing loss in both ears, of the nerve type. We are thinking of having another child, but are afraid that we may have another child with a hearing impairment or a worse defect. Is it possible that the hearing loss could be hereditary?*

A: Approximately one out of every 4,000 live births is a hereditary deaf newborn. A genetic center is the best place to go to receive a thorough examination and evaluation. The risk factors can be explained once genetic information is available.

#22 Q: *I have a four-year-old girl who has just been diagnosed as totally deaf in one ear, with normal hearing in the other ear. I didn't believe the audiologist nor otologist at first because she never complained nor even indicated such a problem. How did it happen that she didn't know it herself; what about school for her, and will she need a hearing aid?*

A: Late detection of a profound hearing impairment in one ear in young children is surprisingly not that uncommon, particularly in healthy alert tots who appear in good physical health. What usually goes on in the mind of a child with such a hearing disorder is the assumption that everybody must hear this way. Normal hearing for her is hearing on one side, in one ear.

She should have no difficulty in school with her hearing problem as long as her hearing is stable in the better ear. However, her seating arrangement should be purposely worked out and discussed with her teachers and her hearing loss explained to them so that they can cooperate with understanding. She should sit in the first row of the classroom with her good ear on the side where the class is.

With your four-year-old child I would certainly not encourage the use of a hearing aid. The psychological and sociological effects at such an early age (and later during early school years) may well produce greater emotional problems for her than any potential benefit she might receive from wearing an aid. As long as she can maintain good grades, good speech and doesn't appear to be suffering, amplification is not my recommendation. Eventually when she is older, she may wish to use a hearing aid for convenience of hearing on that side by use of a CROS type aid (used when an ear is so poor in discrimination that a microphone is placed on the poor side sending sound via a wire over to the better ear).

#23   Q: *I have a child who was diagnosed as deaf at the age of five. She was making speech sounds right from birth, from crying to baby talk. Our pediatrician told us he thought she was retarded and might be best in an institution. I was furious at the thought. How could he have so grossly misdiagnosed a hearing problem?*

A: This is a situation that the majority of parents of deaf children have come upon all too frequently in their early years of discovering their child did not appear to be "normal." A congenitally deaf child is undoubtedly the greatest challenge to the professional world involved in hearing health care. It usually takes time to detect that a child is deaf. It takes so long simply because the hearing loss must be detected by so many people before it can be handled—usually starting with a suspicion by the mother, and then the pediatrician, and then to an otolaryngologist and then to an audiologist. And in between all these visits, you may be stopping in for opinions at one or more local speech and hearing clinics, perhaps through a university. To top it off, you may get differing opinions and that only adds to your confusion. My experience has revealed that parents, particularly mothers, and specifically those mothers who have had other children, are usually correct in their analysis of a hearing problem because they are with that child for so many hours. By the time you get your appointments made and then re-appointments, your child is getting older. Getting to the proper person in the proper facility is all it takes. An evaluation for deafness in the hands of a competent audiologist is not difficult. It only requires getting to him through the channels I have just explained.

Let me point out some additional factors of why it is so difficult to recognize deafness in early infancy. When a child is born deaf (and assuming that the problem is restricted to hearing alone), the infant will cry as normally as the child who hears perfectly. The crying is reflexive. An early diagnosis of deafness by the mother or pediatrician at this age is difficult. It takes a skilled professional. When there are multiple handicaps (such as cerebral palsy, mental retardation, etc.), the diagnosis becomes that much more difficult.

For the first month, an infant usually does little more than cry and eat. Detecting the difference between the child with a serious hearing handicap and the normal hearing child is impossible at this age by mere observation alone. If you rock a severely hard of hearing infant in your arms, there is no way at one month of age to know, as a parent, if that child is not hearing you. You may pop a balloon behind his back and if he fails to jump or become startled, there is a good chance of a potential hearing problem. But for you to detect a problem when there is a *partial* loss of hearing (which could still respond favorably to a hearing aid), your detection of the problem by mere observation alone is highly unlikely. If you clap your hands and your infant jumps from being startled, it does *not* mean that there is no hearing loss, to the dismay of many

115

mothers. A home evaluation that you may perform may greatly mislead you.

In the second month, the hearing infant begins to babble, making sounds because he likes to *hear* them and enjoys the feel of the sounds in his mouth. Still, the hearing handicapped infant produces essentially the same sounds but makes them because they *feel* good, not because they *sound* good. The sounds are not audible to him (assuming that the handicap is severe) or may be greatly distorted if there is some hearing. The infant's babbling may continue for several months. By the fourth month, the hearing infant should be able to localize where a particular sound is coming from in his environment (e.g., right side, left side, from above or below). Somewhere in or around the sixth month, the vocal sounds change. The normal hearing infant starts lalling, that is, producing speech sounds (such as the utterance of "ma-ma") because they attract people or bring about some action or reaction. The infant is finally aware that he can trigger some sort of excitement through his utterances. But this stage of lalling is also the stage where the hearing deficient infant first indicates the nature of his problem. He cannot realize or associate his utterances with behavior because he cannot hear them to make the necessary association. Hence, there is a marked impairment in the development of speech. On the other hand, impaired or delayed speech or language cannot automatically presuppose a hearing problem. All children develop speech at varying rates, some well ahead and some well behind the norm.*

The complaint of "misdiagnosis," as you have put it, is sometimes wailed by new mothers. When a child is far behind in speech development, quick diagnoses are often made, sometimes too hastily, such as brain damage, mental retardation, deafness, autism or aphasia. These or any of a number of other afflictions can account for . delayed speech development. Nonetheless, there should be a wide margin for "normal" allowed, in order to prevent such misdiagnoses.

---

*By 18 months of age, a child usually acquires 10 to 20 spoken words; by age two, about 250 words; by age three, about 1,000 words; and by age five, about 2,000 words.

#24 Q: *My son is hearing impaired and he will be starting public school this fall. Will he need to be in a special class or program or can he be in a regular class with other children?*

A: Many schools throughout the country have integrated hard of hearing children into their program for normal hearing students. I feel it's a shame that more schools have not followed suit. Discrimination against these children, or for that matter any "special child" still exists today, so close to the 21st century. It's unfortunate but that's the way it is. More time will be needed for our world to recognize these human beings as equally sensitive creatures. Generally, the greater (or more obvious) the handicap, the greater the difficulty in adjusting in a public school setting.

I feel that *every* handicapped child should get the opportunity to function in schools for normal children. This accomplishes two things, at the very least. Other children get to realize that the world is not made up of people who have no physical problems and that often, such differences need be no barrier to learning or making friends. In the meantime, the handicapped child gets to realize that in order to make it in the world in which we live, it is imperative to communicate (without fear) with people who do not suffer from the same problems. Frequently, people with common problems prefer being together because when in the company of one another, there is an obvious security in knowing that the other will not pay particular attention to the handicap in a threatening way. Contrary to this, children and adults have the capacity to mock any handicapped individual. Integration of handicapped children into schools for normal functioning students can effectively teach the handicapped person how to better cope with the situations that are bound to come about sometime in his life. Learning how to handle these situations early in life makes for a far more adjusted individual. In the process, children who do not suffer from such afflictions come to realize and better understand the problems these youngsters face.

Many physically handicapped children develop additional problems because they are deprived of the opportunity to make it in a world that consists mostly of people without that

117

particular affliction. Education in an environment with only handicapped children, many with far worse problems than your own child, does not create an environment for education that prepares a child to handle the handicap outside of this particular environment. The child may learn to read and write, but I'm speaking about interpersonal relationships. Special schools have only "special children." Public schools have both "special" and "normal" children. Our world has both. The opportunity for education in a public school is a must. I know people who have been deaf since birth who never attended a school for the deaf. They are well-educated, well-adjusted people living "normal" lives.

If a hearing handicap is so great that your child cannot learn in a public school setting and no program for the hard of hearing exists, then it is important your child be placed in another school setting (even if it's a special school), for no other reason than education.

#25 Q: *Do any government agencies or health insurance programs cover the expense of a hearing evaluation and a hearing aid?*

A: Medicare does not provide coverage for a hearing evaluation that would determine the need for a hearing aid— this is unfortunate. They also do not cover the expense of a hearing aid. It would be a tremendous benefit to all Medicare recipients if they could at least find out if they needed a hearing aid rather than allowing these millions of people to wander uninformed and often end up with a hearing aid that doesn't work, an improper one for their needs, or pay the price of an aid when benefit is not realized. I suspect that by 1980, at least the cost of an evaluation by an audiologist to determine the need for an aid will be covered by Medicare. There is legislation now in Congress proposing this. I would hope that by 1984, Medicare will allow recipients to buy one aid if needed.

Medicaid programs in 26 states* cover the diagnosis of a

---

*California, Connecticut, Illinois, Indiana, Iowa, Kansas, Louisiana, Massachusetts, Minnesota, Montana, Nebraska, Nevada, New Hampshire, New Jersey, New Mexico, hearing disorder and will pay the expenses involved in purchasing a hearing aid. However, the qualifications are rather restrictive.

The Federal Rehabilitation Services Administration, functioning through state departments of vocational rehabilitation, covers the cost of a hearing evaluation if employment related.

The Federal Maternal and Child Health Services, which function through state health departments or crippled children's services, provide financial assistance for children, including evaluation of hearing and a hearing aid (for those who are eligible).

The Veterans Administration covers all the expenses for veterans who have established service connection for their hearing loss.

If you have health insurance, you should contact a representative who can provide you with information on the extent of coverage you have for hearing health care. Many unions cover the total expenses involved in your hearing health rehabilitation, as long as your hearing loss is work related. I have seen dozens of patients with severe high tone hearing loss that resulted from exposure to intense levels of noise at work. In the cases where the employer did not pay for a hearing aid and one was indicated, many consulted an attorney to consider litigation in order to recover the cost of the aid and damages to hearing. In most such cases, the employers suddenly became agreeable to paying for the hearing aid. In the cases where they did not, litigation was initiated, and after their hearing loss was shown to be work related, a substantial amount of compensation was paid to the patient. (Most of these were settlements outside of court.) Since Workmen's Compensation does not cover the expenses, litigation is often warranted and necessary.

There are many prepaid health plans throughout the country that cover hearing evaluations as well as hearing aids. Know what insurance you carry.

New York, North Dakota, Ohio, Oregon, Rhode Island, Utah, Vermont, Virginia, Washington, West Virginia, and Wisconsin.

QUESTIONS ABOUT HEARING AIDS

#26 **Q:** *I was told years ago by a friend that if I got a hearing aid, I could become dependent upon it. Is this true?*

A: Yes and no. The word "dependent" is not a good word for describing a preference for using something that may not be harmful to you. A hearing aid is not a narcotic—that is, something the body grows to depend upon. Are you dependent upon your automobile? Again, the term "dependent" is not appropriate. One is not usually dependent upon a car, although it has become an integral part of our way of life. Some people depend upon medication to stay alive. That's different. But we *can* live without automobiles. Similarly, a hearing aid is something like a Rolls Royce: it simply makes functioning less difficult and thereby makes life a whole lot easier. The body will not grow dependent upon it. However, there may be a great desire to use it frequently because of the great convenience it offers. If it can prevent strain in listening to speech, then I would encourage such "dependence," much like the "dependence" on eyeglasses. If it is available, use it.

#27 **Q:** *I have never worn a hearing aid before this week. I am on a 30-day trial period at the recommendation of my audiologist. I seem to be very conscious that the hearing aid is in my ear. How long will it take before I finally get used to wearing the aid without any particular awareness of it?*

A: I will assume that you are not consciously aware of the aid because it may be an improper one for you. I will often make a recommendation for a specific aid with specific characteristics (such as internal power, frequency emphasis, etc.) and find that it is not the best instrument for that particular patient. Therefore, I will make another recommendation. This is one of the purposes of being on a trial period. None of us are infallible. With so many instruments on the market, there is a good selection available.

Assuming that you do have the proper instrument for your needs, it generally takes anywhere from a few hours to a few months to feel comfortable in putting it on, adjusting the volume when necessary, taking it off, or wearing it without any particular notice of it on the ear. Adjustment to wearing a hearing aid is a very personal thing. It varies from person to person. Much like eyeglasses, it ultimately depends upon the user. My own patients usually find that within a matter of about two weeks, they feel comfortable wearing it. On the other hand, I have seen some patients who never got used to wearing an aid. But I have found that this small group of patients either were fitted with a hearing aid in a department store (and improperly fitted) or had the correct instrument for their hearing loss but were unwilling to accept the fact that they were wearing the aid. This brings up one of the biggest factors in buying an aid or getting used to wearing it.

I have patients ask me frequently, "Do I need a hearing aid?" The moment I am asked that question, I suspect that this patient will have more difficulty in wearing and accepting the aid than the person who comes to me and says, "Look, I've had it! I'm not hearing! I'm missing half of the things that are going on around me. Is there something I can do? Is there a hearing aid I can wear?"

Let's take the patient above who asks if he needs a hearing aid. Sometimes, this type of patient will phrase it more negatively and ask, "You don't think I need a hearing aid, do you?" My answer is immediately, "Of course you don't need a hearing aid!" You should see the patient's eyes light up and a smile fill his face. But then I continue and the smile starts to crack and the eyes begin to droop.

"Nobody ever needs a hearing aid," I explain, "but you do 'need' food. You do 'need' water. You may even 'need' clothing and shelter. But a hearing aid is not imperative for your biological survival. You will make it in life if you never get a hearing aid."

And then the obvious question arises from the patient, "Well, then, are you saying that I shouldn't buy one?"

"No. That's not what I'm saying. I said you do not *need* one. But the fact is that one will most likely make situations of communication far less stressful for you. You should find yourself experiencing less frustration associated with listening. Less anxiety."

Now the patient is confronted, perhaps for the first time, with the realization that *she* or *he* must make the decision as to whether or not to consider an aid. It no longer is *my* decision. I have never strongly urged anyone to purchase a hearing aid. The reason is obvious. If the patient fights the idea of wearing or needing an aid, trying to change his or her mind is a losing battle from the start.

Motivation and desire to obtain help from amplification are absolutely fundamental in the adjustment to wearing a hearing aid. If my patients do not have the determination, a hearing aid will only complicate their lives because they will have tried it at a time that they were not psychologically ready.

So you see what I mean now when I say that adjustment to wearing an aid is a very personal thing. Wearing an aid is intended to make life more pleasurable through making communication less difficult. There is essentially very little physical adjustment to an aid, if it is the proper one.

#28 **Q:** *A friend of mine wears a hearing aid and has been so pleased with it that I decided since I need one, I want to get the same kind. The audiologist told me that he would not recommend that model for me. Why?*

A: There is no "best" make or model hearing aid. What works well on one person may work miserably on another. Of the more than 1,200 models on the market, most of them are fairly good products. The most important part of purchasing a hearing aid is the selection of one by an audiologist after a complete hearing evaluation. The key in fitting a hearing aid with good success is realizing that aids differ in their frequency response, gain and maximum power output. An aid that helps your friend may be impossible for you to tolerate.

#29 **Q:** *I was referred for a hearing aid by an audiologist and I have not gone to get it yet. I am curious about how long it takes to get an aid. What can I expect?*

A: Usually it is not the hearing aid that takes any time at all. Most hearing aid dispensers carry an inventory of hearing aids or they can be ordered and received within 24 to 72 hours.

The earmold is what takes time. On your first visit to a hearing aid office, an impression of your ear canal is taken by pouring soft material into the ear and allowing it to dry. The time-consuming part of this is not the impression, which can take less than five minutes, but sending it to the laboratory to be prepared. This can take from two to ten days. Some dispensers make their own molds which can be ready within a day or two. However, most dealers send them out to be made.

The second visit to the dealer is to fit you with the earmold and a hearing aid. At this time, if any adjustments are necessary on the mold, they are done. Then the aid that was recommended by your audiologist is connected to the mold and put into your ear. Some audiologists do not specify a particular hearing aid to try; they prefer that the dealer select and fit the aid. The audiologist can then evaluate the instrument before it is purchased.

In most cases, the hearing aid is loaned to you on a rental basis for 30 days at a cost of one dollar per day plus the cost of the earmold. This should allow an ample amount of time for you to try the aid and make sure that it is the best instrument for your needs.

#30 Q: *I have been told by my physician that I have a moderate hearing loss in one ear and a mild to moderate loss in the other. He referred me to a hearing aid dealer who tried to sell me two hearing aids. I came in expecting to buy one. Why two?*

A: In the first place, a physician alone is not the best individual to refer you to a hearing aid dealer. This should be the responsibility of an audiologist who routinely refers patients to dealers. If you do not get to see an audiologist through your physician, then you can take the responsibility to find one. If there is no audiologist in your area, then you simply will have to depend upon the word of a well-meaning physician. But the problem is that your physician is not trained to know anything about requesting detailed specifications for a hearing aid to meet your auditory needs, and the salesman dispensing hearing aids receives no formal training in specifications of an aid either.

The situation of fitting one or two ears often appears to have a motive of profit behind it, since the more aids a salesman sells, the greater are his profits. Some information that determines the need for two hearing aids includes:

- How poor is the hearing in your *better* ear? (That is, can you manage with no aid at all on your better ear?)

- What type of loss is present? (Is surgery perhaps possible—did you get a second medical opinion?)

- Can you tolerate the amount of power offered by two aids?

- Are you able to localize the source of sound more easily with the use of one aid than no aid, or do two aids seem to help you locate where sound comes from better than one or none?

- Do you feel "out of balance" with one aid? It is generally a good idea to initially take one hearing aid on a trial (30 to 60 days) basis and use it alternately in the ears, if you do not want two aids. The hearing loss should be quite similar in order to use aids alternately in this way. In any event, hearing aids should be used on trial for at least a month.

#31 Q: *Why did an audiologist try to dissuade me from getting the type of hearing aid that is in the glasses versus the behind-the-ear one?*

A: There are many more advantages to the behind-the-ear type hearing instrument than the eyeglass hearing aid. If you drop your glasses, you risk breaking the hearing aid at the same time. If you wash your glasses you risk eroding the fragile components. On some eyeglass aids, if the aid needs repair, you cannot separate the stems alone and the eyeglasses are also sent away for repair. If you want to rest your eyes by removing your glasses, you are forced to remove your hearing aid also. There is no advantage to wearing eyeglass aids other than for cosmetic purposes. In fact, the life expectancy is less than behind-the-ear aids because of the constant handling of eyeglasses, putting them on, taking them off, dropping them, cleaning, etc. Perspiration is the cause of deterioration in most hearing aids, but the greater the handling, the greater the possibility of damage. Whenever possible, it is a good idea to keep glasses and hearing aids independent of one another.

#32 **Q:** *I wear an ear-level hearing aid in one ear and have developed a habit of pulling my hair over my ear to be sure it is covering the aid. My husband and friends tease me about it. Am I vain?*

   A: Yes, in my opinion. In fact, if your friends are aware that you wear an aid, there seems little need to cover it up. Those who do not see it may become aware of it through your habit. Besides, if the aid is visible to some degree, particularly with new acquaintances, they will be reminded of your hearing difficulty and communicate more carefully with you. I would encourage you to break your habit. Most people accept you wearing a hearing aid—now won't you?

#33 **Q:** *Can a hearing aid further damage my hearing?*

   A: There is research to indicate that a hearing aid with excessive maximum power output can in fact produce greater hearing impairment. Several studies have reported people with hearing disorders who developed additional loss of hearing with the use of certain aids. Removal of the aid in many of these cases allowed the level of hearing to return to what it had been before the aid was used. This is why a proper hearing aid fitted by a competent dispenser is so important.

#34 **Q:** *How can I wear a hearing aid when my ear constantly drains from a chronic infection?*

   A: There is a special hearing aid that is available for amplification with such a problem. It is a bone conduction hearing aid that is the come-on for many hearing aid advertisements claiming "no cords, no tubes, no wires and nothing in the ear." It is not the best instrument available, but for the condition for which it has been designed, it is the only practical solution. The hearing aid receiver fits on the mastoid bone, located behind the ear and is attached to a headband that holds it in place. Some models of bone conduction instruments are designed in eyeglasses. No hearing aid should be worn in the ear if the ear drains from infection. Besides ruining the aid, it can increase the amount of infection.

#35 **Q:** *I have trouble hearing and I'm considering the purchase of a hearing aid through an audiologist, but I never thought to ask if a hearing aid will be able to help me hear better on the telephone. Will it?*

A: There are many factors involved with hearing better on the telephone with the use of a hearing aid. Generally, if you are able to use the phone even with difficulty without a hearing aid, there is a very good chance that with the use of an aid, you will be able to hear much better. At your request, many hearing aids come with an optional "T" switch for telephone use, altering the frequency response of the hearing aid through activation of an electromagnetic induction coil. You merely turn a switch to activate the element. The coil allows better telephone reception by reducing background noise. However, in order for the induction coil to function, your phone must have a pickup coil in the receiver. American Telephone and Telegraph (AT&T) and General Telephone and Electronics (GT&E) throughout the United States have removed pickup coils from receivers in the haste of our rapidly growing technology. GT&E reports already converting 95 percent of their phones to the newer receivers. AT&T has converted about 10 percent (10 million) and is continuing at a rate of approximately two and one-half million per year. The Bell System reports that it would cost one million dollars per year to add the induction coil to the new receivers and fifty million dollars per year for transmission loss due to the coil if used as in the past. In the meantime, the hearing aid industry and telephone companies are in the process of working on an acoustic coupling device that would replace the induction coil, be as effective and cost under fifty cents to purchase.

At the present time this may render the "T" switch rather useless to hundreds of thousands of hearing aid users. However, there are other amplification possibilities available, such as handset receivers equipped with a volume control, or portable telephone amplifiers that can attach to any phone to increase volume.

Information will only be received if you ask for it. Contacting a representative at your local telephone business office may help considerably. However, if you do get a hearing aid with a "T" switch and happen to use a pay phone in some areas, don't be surprised if you cannot hear with it. It may not be your hearing, your aid or a broken telephone, but a receiver without an induction coil. You may wish to contact your local telephone company for information on what receiver you have.

#36　**Q:** *What is the best way to keep the earmold and hearing aid clean? Everybody I have talked to about this has recommended something different, from various solutions to not cleaning it at all. What should I do?*

A: The answer to your question may determine the length of time you maintain your hearing aid in good working order. Hearing aids do not need cleaning by their owners. Should any cleaning be necessary, take it back to the individual from whom you purchased it. He should be able to clean it for you at no expense. The hearing aid simply should never be cleaned because of the danger of ruining it. If for some reason something sticky gets on the aid, a little soap on a very slightly dampened cloth should remove it without a problem. But you shouldn't clean an aid like you'd clean a car! A perfectly dry cloth can remove any moisture that might develop on the aid. Usually no rubbing is necessary, though.

Many people clean hearing aids with all types of solutions, but moisture can destroy an aid. The major reason that hearing aids deteriorate so rapidly is moisture created through perspiration. All aids should remain free from moisture, including steam from cooking, water from showering, sprays for the hair, and excessive perspiration. If heavy work is to be undertaken and a good sweat is going to be worked up, it is always a good idea to remove the aid. Many of my patients who work on jobs that require a lot of physical effort will forget that they have the aid on. After a few weeks of this, they can no longer even read the brand name of the aid on the instrument. Moisture will eventually destroy the aid. In these same patients, if the aid is worn enough while they are overheated and perspiring, the plastic microphone becomes very elastic. At this point, the components inside are likely to be affected.

It is worth keeping in mind that these are fragile instruments. It really does not take much negligence to find yourself back in the hearing aid office for either a repair or a new aid.

As far as cleaning the earmold, bearing in mind what I've just said, a dry cloth can remove any excess wax. If a toothpick, pipecleaner, pin, cotton swab or the like is used to pry wax out of the earmold and/or tubing, there is the risk of pushing the debris further into the mold or tube, or puncturing them.

Many people use earmold solution that is sold for cleaning the earmold. This can be a quick means of buying another aid. Many times, whatever liquid is being used will get into the earmold and work itself up through the tubing and into the aid.

Cleaning the earmold presents no real problems if a few precautions are taken. The earmold should probably be cleaned one or more times a week in lukewarm water and nondetergent soap. BUT DETACH THE EARMOLD FROM THE HEARING AID! This can be done by removing the tubing that connects to the top of the aid. If it is glued, a dealer can assist you in removing it. The cleaning of the mold should be done at night so that it can be allowed to dry overnight and reconnected in the morning. At no time should the mold be connected while it is still damp. For an earmold that is in dire need of cleaning, most hearing aid offices have special equipment for cleaning. It shouldn't cost anything if you are their customer.

#37 Q: *I bought a hearing aid four years ago and it seems to be breaking down so often now that according to my audiologist and hearing aid dispenser, it is best that I buy a new one. How long is the average life of a hearing aid?*

A: The life of a hearing aid has been generally anywhere from three to five years, depending upon the amount of wear and care. This is not to say that it cannot last longer. I have seen patients who have had their aids for ten years or more, some running like a Timex watch that doesn't quit. In cases when the aid still functions and is many years old, there is usually a newer model that can provide more effective amplification. Every few years, manufacturers come up with something that seems to somewhat date hearing aids, like automobiles. This is how industry thrives in the United States. I know that some aids are made better today than five years ago. So there is a certain amount of truth in the greater effectiveness of aids recently put on the market (but do not make the mistake of drawing a gross generalization from this).

In essence, the better you treat your instrument, like a car, the longer you can expect it to last. As would be expected, children go through aids more rapidly than adults for this very reason.

#38 **Q:** *I have worn a hearing aid for years. I recently bought a new one and found that it uses batteries more than twice as fast as the old aid. The new aid uses the same type of batteries but instead of lasting ten days, I only get three days out of one battery. Is something wrong?*

A: No conventional hearing aid should use all the battery power in less than 60 hours.* While some aids give only 60 hours use out of a battery, other aids get 600 hours out of the same battery. It depends upon many factors, including the particular model aid you buy, the amount of power the aid contains, the amount of power you use from the aid, whether or not you are careful and separate the battery from the aid at night when not using the aid, how fresh the batteries may be, and whether or not there may actually be a malfunction (such as a short circuit) in the aid causing excessive battery wear. Let's discuss these in more detail.

Some aids are much more powerful than others. The power varies greatly in different aids, depending upon your need to hear at greater or lesser intensities. Therefore, the

*More than 90 percent of all the aids produced by the top 20 hearing aid manufacturers provide more than 60 battery hours.

more powerful the instrument, the greater the drain on the battery.

Many hearing aids are not affected by the degree to which you turn your volume wheel (particularly less powerful aids). However, you might have stepped up to a more powerful instrument (with push-pull circuitry), whereby battery consumption is affected by changes in your volume setting.

Another important consideration is whether or not you separate the battery compartment (opening it up) from the aid itself. If you turn your aid to the "off" position, you may think that you are not using any power. Many people do not realize that they are in fact using power because the circuit is not broken until the battery is either moved away (by opening the battery compartment) or removed from the aid. Although the amount of wear on the battery is rather minimal if we are speaking of one night, when we look at the picture for many weeks, a good amount of voltage will have been wasted while you perhaps had the aid in your dresser drawer overnight, without separating the battery from the aid. Some new aids have the added convenience of a double notch when pulling out the battery compartment—one to stop battery wear when not in use and another to open it further for replacement of the battery.

Another consideration in battery life is the actual type of battery you buy. There are generally two types that are available. Silver oxide batteries have a shelf life (that is, how long they can remain on a shelf without going dead) of about one year. Mercury batteries have a shelf life slightly longer (about 15 months). Therefore, if a battery is manufactured in Minneapolis in January, it may not leave there until a month later. Then it is shipped to a distributor who might hold the batteries for up to 90 days (now into May). Then he sends them to the retailer who sells them to you. But the retailer may hold them for 90 days without selling them before you make the purchase (which brings us to August). If you buy two packs of batteries (which might be a four to six months' supply), and they happen to be the silver oxide ones, then before you go to use your last battery, you may find that it is dead, because before you used your first battery, the package was already eight months old.

This is not necessarily typical of the shipping process of batteries, but it does occur. I never recommend that my patients buy in excess of two months' supply. Also, it is a good idea to store batteries in a cool, dry place.

It is also entirely possible that you are reusing old batteries if you do not discard used batteries properly. (Take them back to your dealer for him to dispose of since they contain dangerous chemicals.) Batteries will automatically recharge if left sitting long enough. An apparently dead battery may be able to provide another hour or two (sometimes even a day's) worth of power if left to recharge for several days, but don't be misled. The batteries should not be reused even if they recharge because of the likely confusion that could result between which battery is dead and which one is fresh. You can purchase a battery (voltage) tester to check your batteries for about a dollar through most hearing aid dealers.

A final possibility is that the aid is using too much power because it has a malfunction in it. In this case it should be taken back to the dealer from whom you purchased it and he can appropriately test the aid to see if this is the case. Usually, this particular type of problem, if it does happen, occurs with a new aid and is remedied without any expense to you. It is more uncommon to find an aid that you have had for some time developing this malfunction.

#39 **Q:** *My son wears a behind-the-ear hearing aid and lost it on the playground at school this week. I have to spend another four hundred dollars for a new aid and he only had the other one for less than a year. He is 11 years old and usually more responsible but I can't afford to keep buying new ones. What can I do?*

A: I would urge you to take out an insurance policy that is available to you from your hearing aid dealer. Either he has a policy or the manufacturer of the particular aid you buy has a policy to insure you against loss and damage. The rates vary, though. My own patients pay about nine dollars per year for this protection. Those who have had the insurance and have lost the aid know how valuable this policy can be, especially if the aid is for a young child.

#40 Q: *What are the expenses involved in keeping up an aid, including repairs when necessary?*

A: There is essentially minimal expense in keeping up an aid. Perhaps this is fortunate since they are so expensive. Your primary expense will be the battery which generally runs about fifty cents a piece. How many batteries you use will of course determine the expense for you. When we break down the cost of battery wear over time, what we usually find is that for every hour you wear the aid, you use about one cent of energy. Some aids get a full day's use for a cent. Nonetheless, since the cost of living continually goes up (at least since I've been alive), we might anticipate an increase in the future.

Repairs on the aid vary, depending upon what the problem is. Generally, repairs cost from twenty-five to seventy-five dollars. If it runs in excess of this, you may wish to consider buying a new aid if you think you would be buying one in the near future anyway. You must weigh the value of a repair against the investment in a new aid. I have heard of some people paying one hundred fifty dollars for a repair and unfortunately this really should not happen. I don't mean to deny any dealer the right of a profit on a repair, but an exorbitant repair cost is not in your best interest. This does not happen very often, but should you find yourself confronted with this situation, you should feel free to contact your referring audiologist for an opinion.

#41 Q: *There are so many models of hearing aids on the market that I feel bewildered by the array. How am I supposed to know if I get the right one?*

A: Indeed, one could be easily bewildered by the array of hearing aids on the market, but those who are familiar with good aids from dependable manufacturers are in the best possible position to judge what might be most suitable for your needs. The consumer, I'm afraid, must depend upon the knowledge and expertise of the audiologist recommending the aid and the dealer fitting it. You are not expected to know which is best for you any more than you should decide which is the best corrective lens for your vision.

For your protection and benefit, a 30-day trial period is now mandatory in many states when you are purchasing an aid. This trial period allows you enough flexibility so that if you are unhappy with the hearing aid selection, you have the opportunity to try another one, per the recommendation of the audiologist (or dealer), at no additional expense to you. I have had patients that had the best recommendation possible from me, yet they preferred another instrument over my originally specified one simply because it "sounded better." The aids may appear identical on all the sophisticated equipment that we have to test it, but the ultimate test is how it sounds to you once in the ear.

#42 Q: *I am now in the middle of a trial period with my new aid. Although it seems to help me, at times I am bothered by a fullness in my ears and a hollowness in my voice when I wear it. Is this normal?*

A: No. There should be no sensation of fullness nor hollowness. This may be due to the type of earmold that you have. It could be plugging your ear more than you need. In other words, you might be able to manage better with less mass in your ear.

It also could be due to a lack of air getting into your ear canal. Oftentimes, a vent in the earmold resolves this problem. Your dealer can make this adjustment. You should consult him if you suffer from these sensations. He may be able to alter the internal power of the aid or modify the amplification you are getting at some frequencies which might also be causing these sensations. If you do not attain satisfaction from the dealer, you should consult your audiologist who recommended the aid and give him an opportunity to resolve the difficulty. Your complaints are very common and many people are led to believe that this is normal and that they should get used to it. But in fact, this is a problem that can be resolved in 99 percent of my patients and I don't see why it can't be resolved for you.

#43 **Q:** *My otolaryngologist diagnosed me as suffering from Meniere's Disorder about a year ago. One of the symptoms of this condition is my fluctuant hearing. There are days I hear fine and then there are days that I feel like I'm deaf. I can't even hear the telephone ring on my bad days, nor even talk on the phone because I can't hear. My otologist said that it is possible that some day when my hearing drops, it might stay down and not return. In the meantime, when my hearing does go down (sometimes for a few weeks), I need something to help me hear better. Since I would only use a hearing aid for a relatively short time, should I bother getting one?*

A: The symptom of episodic hearing loss with Meniere's Disorder is one of the most frustrating as well as baffling conditions to handle. It is a problem for your otologist and audiologist, as well as for you. I have seen the frustration, anxiety and depression it has caused in many of my patients who suffer from this disorder. A hearing aid can certainly bring some of the hearing problem under control. However, there are people who also lose speech discrimination ability when their hearing drops with Meniere's. This may make the use of a hearing aid less effective but nonetheless it may well prove to be better than nothing at all.

The real question is whether or not the condition is under medical supervision. If not, the purchase of an aid could be very wasteful. In your case, you mention that you are under medical treatment or supervision and hence, the possibility of an aid might be considered.

I prefer to make sure that the condition is somewhat stable before I recommend a hearing aid, mainly because of the severe dizziness, vertigo, nausea and vomiting in addition to a loss of hearing that are associated with this condition. I have seen depression and anxiety build up as a result of this disorder. This is no time to be fitted for a hearing aid. This can go on for weeks and/or months, depending upon how episodic it actually is. Once you are aware of the attacks and are able to handle them with greater control, and your specialist feels you are more stable emotionally and physically, then you can move in the direction of considering amplification.

The choice of a hearing aid is absolutely your own. You must decide if the few times you would wear it would be worth it. It's your investment and therefore ultimately your decision, once it is determined that a hearing aid can help. In your case, with the frustration that your loss of hearing causes you during the attacks of Meniere's, I would encourage you to seek help through the use of a hearing aid. It is important for you to get an aid that has as much flexibility as possible. By this, I mean that some aids have external power adjustments whereby (in addition to your volume wheel), there are tiny adjustment screws for maximum power output (and other possible adjustments including gain and frequency response). This will allow you or your hearing aid dealer (or audiologist) to make whatever adjustments are necessary when your hearing does decrease during an episode of Meniere's. As you say, sometimes there is a minor loss in hearing while other times there is a rather significant decrease. The aid can then be adjusted internally according to your needs.

#44 **Q:** *My father suffered a stroke which caused paralysis. He also experienced a hearing loss at the same time. He cannot leave the house so I am wondering what we might be able to do to get him a hearing aid without resorting to a door-to-door solicitor.*

A: I assume that your father does have a hearing loss and that this is not the result of some other condition that might be secondary to a stroke, such as auditory agnosia or more commonly, auditory aphasia. These are conditions that are recognized as expressive problems where the person hears you, but cannot process the information correctly, and therefore appears to have a hearing problem.

I also assume that your father has been seen by an audiologist and that he has recommended the purchase of a hearing aid. Audiologists, like physicians, can make home visits. I recommend that your audiologist set up a referral for your father to be seen at a convenient time by a hearing aid dealer. This can be done very easily if you merely contact your audiologist. This way, your father can get the best rehabilitative care available.

#45   **Q:** *What criteria can I use to determine if the hearing aid dispenser I go to is good at his work and will serve my best interests?*

A: Use the same criteria that you use to determine if your physician and audiologist are good at their work, whatever that criteria might be. If you have a lot of confidence in your otologist and audiologist, I'd feel safe in trusting their judgment in referring you to a dealer who they have found from their experience to be dependable, to provide good service and to have reasonable prices.

It otherwise would be rather difficult to find out who in the community is competent. You might turn to somebody who has bought a hearing aid in the past and who could recommend the same dealer to you, but here you are depending upon the judgment of one person (not part of a hearing health team) who might have happened into a good purchase. You would benefit much more from the experience of professionals who routinely work with various hearing aid dispensers.

#46   **Q:** *I have seen several television advertisements by a particular company that has a large nationwide department store chain. They are promoting their hearing aids, at supposedly reduced prices with great warranties. Is it okay to buy from them?*

A: There are many large chain stores similar to the one you mention that advertise this way. Many of them have huge catalogues with thousands of items to choose, from clothes to tires and anything in between. You might have made a purchase from such a company many years ago, other than a hearing aid, and find that the product is still in fairly good shape. It may surprise you, but the chances are that their hearing aids are relatively good also. However, the serious problem with these companies is not the quality of the product, but the quality of the service of those who sell the product.

These types of chain companies buy from one major manufacturer who makes hearing aids under another brand name. This manufacturer then simply stamps the name of the department store onto the aids that go to them (instead of putting their own brand name on it). For all intents and purposes, the aids are quite good. However, the selection and variety of aids is greatly restricted to whatever models that this one manufacturer produces. If you want a specific model and they don't carry it, you are out of luck. Chances are they will attempt to sell you one anyway.

The real problem is that these salesmen are not trained nor equipped to test, evaluate and assess your hearing loss. Should you have some pathology of the ear that should receive medical attention, they are under no obligation to refer you for medical help.

That is why when you purchase a hearing aid, it should be done by referral through an audiologist. Large department stores do not work with hearing health professionals. Their interest is in sales.

#47 **Q:** *I was referred for a hearing aid by an audiologist. He said that my hearing was decreased in both ears and I have come to recognize this to be the case only recently. He said that I could benefit from an aid in both ears since they have about the same amount of loss. I cannot afford two aids at this time so he recommended one aid that I could alternate as I'd like between the ears. This of course would require two separate earmolds, one for each ear. I have been using the aid as he suggested but I still have trouble understanding speech. What else can be done?*

A: Other than the purchase of another aid, there is little that can be done to actually help you hear better. You could take up speechreading, which would not help you to hear better, but would compensate for diminished hearing acuity. It sounds like two aids would be better than one in your case and one is certainly better than none. As long as one ear still suffers from a hearing impairment, the best aid in the world will not solve your hearing difficulty.

I have found with my own patients who suffer from a loss of hearing in both ears (but only have one aid) that if you are really perceptive about the listening situations with which you will be confronted, you can predict which ear will do more of the listening. In so doing, you can be prepared for that situation by wearing the one aid in the appropriate ear. For instance, if you are to have lunch with one person, you would naturally have them seated on your aided side. If you are taking a long trip in the car, and you are the passenger, you would want the one aid on your left ear, amplifying the voice of the driver, and not on the right side, amplifying traffic sounds. But if you are part of a round-table discussion, one aid on either ear will not really be sufficient. The same problem would arise if you were trying to communicate in a car with noisy children, or in your living room with the television playing loudly. The situation of communication increases in difficulty with an increase in the environmental noise when wearing one aid. More noise can be tolerated with two aids (like two ears) because of the phase difference between the ears. You will notice the greatest benefit from the single aid in situations with the least amount of competing noises.

You could perhaps get a better idea of what I mean by two ears helping you more than one ear in a noisy situation by the following demonstration. Even if you have normal hearing, this will work. Turn a radio or television on (preferably a radio with music), and turn the volume up as loud as you normally do. Plug one ear with your finger so that you hear from one ear only. Have somebody ask you questions from several feet away in a low voice and see if you can understand them. The chances are if you do understand them, it will be with great difficulty because two ears work together to bring out the foreground message while reducing the background level of noise. One hearing aid cannot compensate for two ears nor can one good ear compensate for two. You may be informed that two microphones on one hearing aid (known as directional) can compensate for two ears. They cannot.

A fundamental problem that most people with one hearing aid and a bilateral hearing loss experience is a great tendency to turn up the volume. In doing this they are actually trying to get two ears' worth of hearing out of one aid, and it cannot be done. By using a second aid, you may be quite surprised to find that you actually wear the first aid at a lower volume setting than when it was your only aid.

#48 **Q:** *I have worn a hearing aid for years and am puzzled by how well I can hear on the telephone, even under poor listening conditions. Yet even under better listening conditions, I have difficulty hearing people in conversation. Why?*

A: This really is not so puzzling when we look at the mechanics of what is happening. You obviously have a telephone switch on your hearing aid or you would not hear better on the telephone than in face-to-face conversation. The telephone switch activates a magnetic coil within the hearing aid that creates a magnetic field around the hearing aid and telephone when in contact with the phone receiver. While doing this, it eliminates thousands of frequencies in the room that you do not need and focuses in on a very narrow range of frequencies that are carried by the telephone. (The telephone frequencies are usually between 1500 Hz and 2500 Hz.) The frequencies that are eliminated are those that are present when you turn your aid back to the microphone position for normal listening. The success you have with the aid on the phone is largely because you are hooking up one mechanical device to another (aid to phone). Unfortunately, the human voice cannot be rigged up so neatly to a hearing aid because there are many more frequencies being transmitted by the voice than through the phone. Hence, much more extraneous noise will be present in face-to-face conversation (because more frequencies are present) than when using the phone.

#49 **Q:** *Should I wear my hearing aid all the time?*

A: I suggest to my patients that they treat their hearing aid much like glasses—wear it when you feel you can benefit. I wear my glasses in situations when I fully realize I do not benefit from them, yet I do not remove them. It would be more inconvenient for me to take them off than to simply continue wearing them. Most people who wear hearing aids do the same. At bedtime, naturally, they should be removed. It isn't customary for people to sleep with a hearing aid on any more than eyeglasses. But occasionally I have found patients who do go to bed with their hearing aids on, so that if their child cries in the middle of the night, the cry will be heard. The ear deserves a rest from amplification unless there is a definite purpose in wearing it while sleeping.

#50   **Q:** *Will my hearing aid solve all my hearing problems?*

   A: I recommend that if this question persists for any length of time, you reread this book for the answer.

Chapter VII
CASE HISTORIES OF HEARING PROBLEMS

Since I have been practicing audiology, I have come upon many interesting cases of hearing loss. The following cases are a few outstanding ones that I feel are informative as well as interesting.

CASE 1: THE COTTON SWAB NEUROTIC

Mr. J.J. was seen by me about six months ago. He was a very nice and friendly gentleman of 72, but a bit forgetful. He had reclined into his favorite chair for television viewing late one night and reached for a cotton swab as he became engrossed with the action in front of him. Mr. J.J. had massaged his ears for years with cotton swabs, not that they needed cleaning, he said, but it just "felt good."

Cotton swabs often act to push earwax deeper into the ear canal rather than removing it. It may jam wax up against the eardrum and create severe pain, rupture of the drum and/or loss of hearing.

As Mr. J.J. sat viewing the television and rubbing the cotton swab in his ear, the telephone rang beside him. It momentarily startled him, but he quickly answered it, putting the receiver to his ear—but he forgot to remove the cotton swab first.

At the time I saw Mr. J.J., his pain was under control after treatment by one of the otologists in the clinic. The cotton swab had rapidly passed through the eardrum, broken the delicate middle ear bones and lodged in the inner ear structure (the cochlea). Rupture of the inner ear allowed the contained fluid to escape, producing instant and permanent deafness in that ear. The hearing loss was so complete that a hearing aid could not have been of any benefit.

Although such a hearing loss is not reversible, it certainly is preventable. The experience of Mr. J.J. is one that has happened to many people. More frequently, patients have less loss of hearing with less traumatization to the ear than Mr. J.J. Most cotton swab accidents rupture the eardrum and may jolt the middle ear bones or displace them. This often results in needed surgery to correct the hearing impairment which is usually mild (unless the damage extends to the inner ear). But a cotton swab need go no further than the eardrum to produce a total loss of hearing. If a cotton swab hits the eardrum, the middle ear bones can become severely traumatized (since the eardrum is connected to the first middle ear bone—the malleus). This shock can carry through to the third tiny bone which can be pushed into the inner ear.

For all cotton swab neurotics like Mr. J.J., nothing smaller than an elephant's foot should ever enter the outer ear canal.

CASE 2: SWIMMER'S EAR

Diana, a child of eleven, was brought into the ear, nose and throat clinic because of an infection in the outer ear canals. It was summer again and Diana was becoming a frequent visitor of the clinic. Due to her many hours in the water while swimming, an infection had occurred in her ear canals. Although most people are unaffected by such exposure, Diana was prone to developing what has become known as "swimmer's ear." The medical term for her condition is actually external otitis (or otitis externa). Many people who live in tropical climates or in areas with very humid summers have a certain susceptibility to this condition.

Diana's ear canals had swelled up from the infection, but

not enough to close off the ear and create a hearing loss (although it can happen). In cases when the canal does swell up and produce hearing loss, the loss is only temporary and is remedied as soon as the swelling diminishes. "Swimmer's ear" is actually a misleading term for Diana's condition because it could have been caused in other ways. Many people who develop otitis externa never go swimming. It can be caused by excessive washing, perspiration, use of eardrops, irritation in the ear canal from removal of foreign bodies, allergies, exposure to fluid that may be draining from the middle ear cavity, or from any systemic disease.

Diana was seen by an otologist who treated the bacterial growth around the eardrum and within a matter of a few days, the infection cleared up completely. Occasionally such a condition becomes chronic, producing constant drainage, swelling and infection. Due to her excessive exposure to moisture, Diana was encouraged to wear earplugs, which proved to be effective for her.

In a recent study done on gerbils, otitis externa was intentionally produced. The animals were found to be so sensitive from outer ear canal traumatization that they died. This certainly is not to suggest that otitis externa kills humans—it doesn't. But immediate medical attention is recommended to prevent complications.

CASE 3: FOREIGN BODIES IN THE EAR CANAL

Mark was a farm child, seven years of age. He complained of an earache while in school one day and was seen by the school nurse. She looked in his ear and did not see much other than a small accumulation of wax in one ear. She performed a hearing test which indicated normal hearing in one ear and a very minor hearing loss in the other ear containing the wax. A note was sent home with Mark, reporting these findings and suggesting that the parents consult a physician. Mark's mother read the note and disregarded it since Mark had not complained of any hearing loss.

But Mark's ear began to hurt again about two days later while at school and he saw the school nurse for the second time.

143

Again she sent Mark home with a note urging that he be seen by a physician. Mark's mother at last complied and they consulted their family physician who referred Mark to the ear, nose and throat clinic.

Mark was seen first by an otologist who immediately removed the accumulation of wax. Normally, the removal of wax is not terribly uncomfortable—but Mark found that it hurt. In the middle of the wax a grain of wheat was discovered. Since the grain was based in wax and far enough into the ear to receive warmth—it sprouted. When the root began to dig into the skin of the ear canal, it caused the discomfort that Mark complained of. The grain was removed without complications and there was no hearing loss.

I have seen children in my office for apparent hearing loss or ear infection produced by any of a number of items inserted into the ear canal. These items have included almost anything from food to live insects, pencil erasers, paper, cherry pits, marbles, crayons, buttons, jewelry and miniature toys. There is little doubt in my mind that if the ear canal were any larger, we might find even more intriguing artifacts.

The length of time that the grain of wheat had remained in Mark's ear was estimated to be three months—at which time he had helped his father with the wheat harvest. But fortunately for Mark, his personal harvest came early that year.

CASE 4: SNOWMOBILES WITH DANGEROUS NOISE LEVELS

Alex was a young man of 22 who was seen in my office in 1970. His primary complaint was that of apparent decreased hearing acuity noticed particularly within the past few weeks.

A case history revealed no family history of hearing problems, no ear infections nor earlier complaints about a hearing problem. Test results showed the type of high frequency hearing loss bilaterally that is typical of noise exposure. Inquiry as to what exposure he might have been subjected to revealed only one possibility—snowmobiles. He claimed that he drove a snowmobile frequently during the winter months, usually six months out of the year. His father owned a farm in upstate New York where he and his family would spend hours driving across miles of snow in the wilderness. Since I also was a fan of snowmobiles, I was well aware of the dangerous noise levels that are constantly present while driving these machines.

Alex reported that he had also been involved in racing snowmobiles. Races would often last up to eight hours, not including the trials and preparation that could easily push exposure to twelve hours. He stated that he had been involved with snowmobiles for three years and racing them for only the past winter. He said that at the end of an eight-hour race, he literally could not hear some people talking to him.

I urged Alex to abstain from all such exposure for at least one week, until he could return for more hearing testing. Frequently, if there is a temporary threshold shift in hearing as a result of exposure to noise, the hearing should start to return to the former level of hearing within 48 hours.

Upon his return to my office one week later, there in fact was an increase in his hearing in the higher ranges but nonetheless, evidence of a slight high tone loss. I informed Alex that it would be unlikely that further hearing would be restored, and, should there be additional exposure to noise in the future, he would be a prime candidate for further hearing deterioration. His hearing loss could become more and more acute with less recovery in that 48-hour period following noise exposure.

The mechanism for hearing is like a rubber band: it stretches and returns to nearly its former shape, stretches and returns, stretches and returns less to its former shape, stretches and returns less . . . and less . . . and less . . . and then one day it stretches and breaks. Any human mechanism cannot be continually overtaxed and abused without eventually paying the price.

Recent research has shown that snowmobiles produce as much as 136 dB of noise. Such exposure must be considered extremely hazardous for *any* length of time. In addition, at snowmobile races, drivers and spectators alike are exposed to no less than generally 80 dB and as much as 108 dB (94 dB average) over an eight-hour period. OSHA reports that this level of exposure should never exceed four hours. Hearing evaluations on the drivers of these racing machines have revealed in one study that all 21 drivers suffered significant high frequency hearing impairment with thresholds that may well never shift back to their former level of hearing acuity prior to racing—leaving permanent hearing loss. But this can be prevented by utilizing ear protection.

Alex was fortunate that he experienced only a temporary loss in hearing and that much of his hearing did return. Many people are far less fortunate than Alex.

CASE 5: DECOMPRESSION

John had been scuba diving and developed a hearing loss in both ears as a result of ascending too rapidly from lower depths of the ocean. I saw him first 24 hours after the episode at which time he was experiencing some pain in the right ear.

Scuba diving and skin diving are becoming very popular sports, and as with many sports, there are definite hazards to be aware of. John did not allow for sufficient decompression as he swam toward the surface of the ocean. His middle ear could not adjust to the rapid change in air pressure, resulting in a rupture of the right eardrum and potential damage to the delicate middle ear bones due to the force of water into the middle ear cavity of his right ear. As a result, he had a mild loss of hearing, of the conductive (operable) type, in his right ear.

His left ear also revealed a mild conductive hearing loss, produced by a eustachian tube malfunction brought on by what is known as ear squeeze (lack of middle ear pressure). The middle ear pressure in the left ear was evidently so great that the stapes (the tiny bone that enters the inner ear) had been greatly displaced but did not actually break. The displacement caused a distortion in the fluid-filled chambers of the inner ear (cochlea) resulting in a permanent high frequency hearing loss.

Within two weeks, John fully recovered from the conductive hearing problems in both ears and was left with the high tone hearing loss in the left ear. The loss was far enough above the critical speech reception range so that John was not even aware that he had a loss of hearing.

CASE 6: DANGEROUS NOISE WITHIN INCUBATORS FOR NEWBORNS

Karen was an infant that was born prematurely. She was delivered by cesarean nearly three and one-half months earlier than expected. She was observed from birth very closely, being quite tiny and underweight as most premature babies are. Karen was placed inside an incubator that was considered imperative for her survival. She remained in her synthetic environment 24 hours a day for several months, until it was felt that the risk of infection had decreased sufficiently.

However, a peculiar thing was noticed in her third month. Karen, although wide-eyed and alert at birth, seemed to be ignoring sounds in her environment that she earlier had responded to. An audiologist was consulted and measurement of Karen's hearing was undertaken. A hearing loss was noted as a result of exposure to the noise emissions from the incubator. The level of sound measured in excess of 80 dB. The apparent hearing loss that Karen suffered was primarily in the lower frequencies which corresponded to the frequencies coming from the electric motor and fan of the incubator. Considering that infants remain in these incubators for many months, and some for more than a year, they are particularly vulnerable creatures. Karen experienced permanent hearing loss. It could have been prevented.

These incubators are still in wide use today. There is considered to be a lack of quantitative evidence that they can in fact produce hearing loss. It is not necessary to see radiation to know that it can be dangerous. Hearing loss is not visible to the eye. Whether we speak of incubators or any other noise-emitting product, it is important to establish and enforce regulations. Karen's story is just one of thousands. She has been deprived of her hearing in part, without her first having experienced the beauty of it.

CASE 7: HEARING AID AT THE WRONG FREQUENCY

Frank was an experienced hearing aid user who lost a considerable amount of hearing by exposure to gunfire during

World War I. As a veteran, he had been covered by the Veterans Administration.

Frank was pushing 90 years of age but was very alert and witty. He had just been fitted with another hearing aid and seemed pleased. However, when he got home, he found that he heard voices—people talking. Knowing that there were no neighbors for at least 100 yards, he couldn't figure out what the problem was. He returned the next day to the audiologist at the V.A. facility who tested the aid without finding any type of malfunction. Frank insisted that he was not crazy and that this was not a joke. At the risk of embarrassment, Frank suggested that he would take the aid back if they didn't believe him. Further investigation by the audiologist as to Frank's actual complaints brought to the surface some vital facts. Frank only complained of the problem while using the instrument at home. In addition, he would hear the word "over" more than any other word from a voice that was not in his house. It was discovered that Frank's neighbor owned a ham radio operator's set and was often broadcasting at night when the signals were much stronger and capable of traveling considerably further.

A hearing aid should not be affected by such broadcasting, but occasionally a circuit will be capable of picking up frequencies that it isn't intended to. Some hearing aid users have complained of receiving radio station interference, police and other emergency vehicle communications. It's a fluke. It isn't supposed to happen.

A hearing aid may well pick up frequencies other than what the factory specifications might indicate. Frank was provided with another hearing aid and is reported doing quite well.

CASE 8: ACUPUNCTURE TREATMENT FOR HEARING LOSS

Billy, age eight, and his mother were seen in my office to discuss a pretreatment audiogram. Billy's mother had arranged an acupuncture treatment program for him at one of the local centers for acupuncture. Billy's hearing loss was in the mild sensorineural range in both ears. He was wearing two aids that seemed to compensate extremely well for his hearing loss. Billy's mother felt that if there was even a remote possibility for medical treatment to improve his hearing, she wanted to try it. She seemed more concerned than Billy about his hearing loss. He seemed to be managing quite well.

Billy's mother set him up in a program comprising 30 acupuncture treatments. She wanted me to evaluate his hearing before, during and after a series of treatments. The initial visit to this particular acupuncture center was fifty dollars. Each subsequent visit ran thirty-five dollars. The total investment was expected to be eleven hundred dollars if Billy underwent all 30 treatments. However, if after 10 treatments there would be no recognizable improvement in hearing, the treatments were to stop. This happened to be one of the more inexpensive programs available.

With Billy and his mother in my office, I explained that there was absolutely no documented successful treatment for hearing disorders through the use of acupuncture. I explained that acupuncture had apparently been successful in the treatment of other physical conditions, but this should not be confused with the disappointment that exists with acupuncture as applied to hearing. The patient's mother insisted that she knew of increased hearing acuity and that such treatment was successful for some people. She showed me an article that appeared in a major newspaper about how such treatment had benefitted many hearing impaired people in the Washington, D.C. area, at one of the large acupuncture centers there. I explained that this simply is not the case and that the newspaper was not reporting accurate information. I informed her that acupuncture for hearing loss was at best experimental and that I sincerely believed she would be losing her investment if she proceeded. In addition, she would be creating false hopes for both herself and Billy.

She was insistent and refused to accept my recommendation. She desired that her son go through the acupuncture treatment program at any cost—and he did.

I saw Billy and his mother again at mid-treatment after he had been through 10 sessions. My first question was directed to

Billy. "Do you think that you hear any better now?" I inquired. "I don't know," he responded. His mother stated that she knew he was hearing better because Billy did not ask to have statements repeated so frequently. I asked Billy if he felt that this was the case for him and he nodded in agreement. However, the audiogram at this time revealed absolutely no change in his hearing. Therefore, there was again no documented evidence of acupuncture having any physical effect upon hearing. Yet the child and mother recognized some sort of improvement in hearing. How?

I asked Billy to have a seat in the waiting room while I discussed the matter with his mother. I explained to Billy's mother that the complex psychological factors at work here set up an illusion that could easily intrigue the best research psychologist; what appeared to be an improvement in hearing was not really so.

The investment of such a substantial amount of money creates high expectations for success. Certainly it would be hoped that after having already spent over four hundred dollars, there would be some improvement in hearing. But there was no physical improvement.

What accounted for Billy's apparent improvement in hearing was his ability to listen better, and in so doing, actually hearing better in the process. This can be done by observing the lip and speech movements more carefully, paying closer attention to the context of what is being discussed and even perhaps turning the hearing aid up louder. She found it extremely difficult to accept my explanation because she still fostered unreal expectations.

Billy continued with additional treatments against my recommendation. The same situation happened again in my office after the 20th and the 30th treatments. There was no measurable improvement.

Billy's mother suffered great disappointment and depression after about five weeks, when Billy returned to his leisure listening habits and it became evident that what had appeared to be an improvement in hearing, unfortunately, was not. Billy seemed relatively unaffected by the entire matter, well adjusted to his hearing loss and benefitting from the use of his hearing aids.

About three months later, I saw them both again in my office after Billy began rejecting his hearing aids. His mother wanted to know what could be done to correct the situation now.

His mother had been very unsupportive of Billy wearing his aids. She had encouraged him to grow his hair longer to cover them up, making him more conscious of them altogether. Billy said that the kids at school were teasing him about the aids, but his mother reported that this was not the case at all. Billy said that he did not want to wear the aids anymore. I agreed to this since I felt that if I pushed the situation, I would create more resistance from him. I was certain that with Billy's hearing loss and lack of amplification, it would not be very long before he would discover how beneficial the aids really were.

His mother's inability to cope with her son's hearing loss had created a hearing problem. In addition, it was likely that there now was an emotional problem related to the hearing problem.

His mother phoned me one month later. She said that she had moved Billy to the front row of his class as I had suggested some time earlier and although that did help him hear better for a time without his aids, he finally went back to wearing them and was much happier. She said that she also was happier because she now realized how much the aids truly did help him.

CASE 9: A CASE OF RINGING EARS

One of the most frequent complaints associated with hearing problems is tinnitus (ringing in the ears). Tinnitus is often a symptom of some other organic problem including potential hearing loss. It is often a kind of warning signal.

Alma was seen in my office because she had been suffering from annoying tinnitus for four months without any relief. She was 43 years of age and although she had a slight hearing loss in the higher frequencies in both ears, it was nothing unusual for her age. She denied having been exposed to noise in the past (which very often can produce tinnitus). A search back to the time when the ringing began revealed that she was being treated by a physician for a problem unrelated to hearing. It was suggested that she take aspirin to control her discomfort during treatment of her other condition. She did. In fact, she took an average of 13 aspirins per day, approaching nearly 100 per week. Her actual tinnitus appeared approximately during the treatment for her other problem.

Alma was put on a non-aspirin pain controller by her physician and the tinnitus slowly diminished within a few weeks.

Aspirin is a known ototoxic medication and can do damage to many organs, including the hearing mechanism. A six-month follow-up on Alma revealed that the tinnitus was greatly reduced, but still present.

I had another patient with the same complaint as Alma. Sam had bothersome tinnitus for many years. He thought that he might have a hearing loss. His hearing evaluation indicated a high frequency loss similar to Alma's. Again, this was nothing so unusual for a man of 52. He spent most of his years as an accountant in a quiet business office and denied any exposure to loud noises. Hence, as in Alma's case, there appeared to be no noise exposure that might have produced the high tone loss and tinnitus. His case history revealed that he had been treated on and off for many years for alcoholism. I asked him if he still partook of the beverage and he said that he never drank more than one can of beer an hour. Obviously, Sam was still experiencing heavy drinking and was doing what he could to control it.

Like aspirin, caffeine, nicotine, or quinine, alcohol can produce tinnitus. Any of these in excess can be very lethal to the hearing mechanism.

Sam said that he had been drinking most of his life and only recently experienced the ringing ears. But the amount of time it takes to produce tinnitus and the amount of ototoxic chemical ingested varies greatly from person to person.

I suggested that he abstain from alcohol intake for a few days but I knew that would be like asking him to lose 50 pounds by midnight. He said that he'd try if that appeared to be the cause—but he didn't.

152

I received a phone call from him about two months later and he reported that he didn't touch a drop to drink for four days because his wife threatened to leave him and take the children. He reported that he did notice that there was a decrease in his ringing and wanted to know if somehow it could be treated.

He was seen by an otologist who put him on a vasodilator (nicotinic acid), but it did not prove effective. Perhaps the most fundamental reason it did not prove effective was that he returned to his drinking habits. In addition, there is no known medical treatment for the elimination of tinnitus. The best treatment is no doubt eliminating whatever it is that is causing the tinnitus, provided that the cause can be determined.

CASE 10: LABYRINTHITIS

Mr. A. was seen in my office one morning for a hearing evaluation. He had developed a sudden hearing loss in one ear during the middle of the night. He reported that he awoke with a pressure in his right ear. He attempted to get out of bed but experienced great dizziness and loss of balance. His wife assisted him back to bed at which time he realized he could not hear out of his right ear.

Mr. A. had a total loss of hearing in one ear, but claimed to have heard well prior to the incident. He was seen by an otolaryngologist that morning, and a diagnosis of acute labyrinthitis was made. This condition is not uncommon and can involve severe vertigo, dizziness, and/or loss of hearing usually in one ear only. Labyrinthitis is the result of a vascular or metabolic condition about which little is known today. There does exist treatment for the condition but whether or not the treatment is at all effective is questionable due to the fact that without any treatment whatsoever, many such cases of labyrinthitis recover completely without any recurrence. Very similar to Meniere's Disorder, present treatment consists of intravenous shots of niacin (nicotinic acid) and histamine which act to expand the blood vessels so that more blood can circulate throughout the body, including through the ear. In theory, this vasodilation nourishes the inner ear, but unfortunately, research evidence is not at all conclusive on the actual medicinal benefit from these treatments.

Control of the symptoms of dizziness or vertigo is often successful through appropriate medication that is prescribed.

Since essentially little is known about labyrinthitis, treatment is difficult. The cause of labyrinthitis is not known although there are theories. The condition can be episodic with recurring attacks or a one-time attack only.

Mr. A. experienced one attack only. He was given no treatment at all and within six weeks, his hearing was back to nearly normal (with a remaining high frequency hearing loss in the right ear). Many patients are given the treatment mentioned above and their hearing has returned. And then there are cases that do or do not get treatment and their hearing never returns. It is quite unpredictable but generally safe to say that if there is no improvement in hearing within two months, there may not be any future restoration.

During Mr. A.'s six-week battle with labyrinthitis, his hearing slowly improved almost day by day. His ability to understand speech improved also, from initially no speech discrimination ability to finally 90 percent. He has not experienced another attack since that time and apparently is doing well.

CASE 11: SUDDEN ONSET OF
HIGH FREQUENCY HEARING LOSS

This case is about Darryl, 42 years old, married and a long-time employee for a telephone company in Los Angeles. He enjoyed working as a poleman, which entailed climbing high telephone poles and working around high-voltage power lines. He enjoyed the thrill of working on the edge of disaster—and he met it one day.

It was a Thursday afternoon when I saw Darryl in my office, one week after he had accidentally grabbed hold of a live, hot wire as he was working from low on a telephone pole. Considering that he was fortunate just to be alive, he voiced very few complaints. Nonetheless, he thought that he might have lost some hearing.

Testing revealed that he had lost some hearing indeed.

The pattern of his hearing loss was remarkable. His hearing was normal through the lower and mid frequencies and at precisely 3000 Hz (area of highest pitched consonants), no hearing existed at all.

His complaints weren't that he couldn't hear, but that he felt "sort of plugged up," in addition to sensing that some sounds appeared a bit muffled. These are common complaints by people who suffer from high tone hearing loss.

What was most unusual about Darryl's loss of hearing was the way in which there was almost no delineation between the point where he heard all right and the point where he had no hearing at all. An analogy would be trees in a forest catching fire and trying to figure out where the trees were that were unaffected. What you'd see are sections where the fire became less and less intense until finally there would be trees that were not harmed at all. You would not find trees totally destroyed next to trees that were thriving, totally untouched by the fire. But in fact, analogous to this, Darryl's hearing loss was intriguing. It was not a gradual deterioration.

The extremely high voltage had evidently burned out or destroyed hair cells within the cochlea where electrical activity occurs.

I informed Darryl that there is no hearing aid that could compensate for his hearing loss since the damage was nearly beyond the critical range for speech reception. We do not have to hear much beyond 3000 Hz to catch what is being said, although harmonics of speech do occur much higher and add to what we know as the "quality" of speech.

What Darryl sensed was a loss in the quality of sound rather than a loss of hearing for speech. Had the damage extended down further into the range below 3000 Hz, he would have been far more aware of a hearing loss.

Darryl was seen several months later. He had no change in hearing and was managing very well.

CASE 12: SUDDEN DEAFNESS IN BOTH EARS

Larry was a veteran with no history of any outstanding hearing loss. He was planning to make the Army a career, but found that he needed extra income to help in the support of his foster children and a new baby on the way.

Larry landed an evening job, moonlighting in a gas station. He had worked there for quite some time when one evening a main gas line leaked. Larry, unaware of this, lit a cigarette and the last thing he recalled was an explosion. The station was destroyed by fire. Larry suffered burns over 90 percent of his body.

After regaining consciousness, he discovered that all the joints in his body except his right arm had frozen and locked up on him. This is often one of the secondary effects of severe burns.

He experienced no hearing impairment from the accident and was able to communicate with his physicians, surgeons and rehabilitators about his condition. Within the first week after the accident, he took a turn for the worse and was administered neomycin as a lifesaving measure. The drug is a known ototoxic medication and has caused deafness in many people. But the question in Larry's case was not one of potential deafness, but of survival for this 27-year-old veteran.

The neomycin produced deafness for Larry, but apparently saved his life. The damage to his hearing was so complete that in one ear a hearing aid could be of no benefit. The other ear responded somewhat to a hearing aid, allowing him to detect only the presence of speech, but not to understand it.

A colleague of mine was consulted and worked with Larry's rehabilitation. She taught him to speechread and make the most of the aid that she had recommended.

Larry had always prided himself on how well he could diagnose engine trouble by listening to the lull of the motor. Obviously, this was to be no more. In fact, things did not look terribly favorable for Larry. He went through the amputation of three fingers on one hand and two on the other. His body resisted many of the skin grafts, and some of the surgical procedures to unlock his joints had failed. In addition, his new little son had been born while he was still under intensive care.

Perhaps quite justifiably so, Larry went into a state of depression.

He found it difficult to smile anymore with a future that looked so dim. But in time, over a few months, he was beginning to recover from the burns, his joints were responding to surgery and he was learning to speechread. My colleague had seen a remarkable improvement in Larry's speech within the first two months.

To pick his spirits up, he was informed that he could take his first weekend pass home to see his wife and new baby. Once home, he realized that he could no longer hear the voice of his wife, nor would he ever get to hear the laughter of his child. Larry felt extreme isolation which only intensified his underlying depression. He felt removed and separate from the family that meant everything to him.

Of all his problems, including the severe burns and scars, the amputations, the inability to move his joints and the constant pain, Larry revealed that none compared to the consequences of not being able to hear.

He found that without human communication, there was a terrifying void in his life—a void that surpassed pain. He said that his loss of hearing was like a profound emptiness, the result of a near-total inability to hear the spoken words of people he knew and loved.

Considering the physical, mental and emotional barriers that Larry faced, he needed an overwhelming amount of determination to survive.

He had determination, though. And he had much support from his family and the Veterans Administration. Larry slowly came out of his depression as he found it easier to speechread. His body was responding at last to skin grafts and surgery on his joints. He was also allowed to spend his weekends with his family.

After more than a year in the V.A. hospital, Larry was able to walk again and speechread remarkably well. He was on his way to rehabilitation.

The V.A. helped him through drafting school so that he could develop a career and become less dependent.

Larry is now a draftsman and deafness is no longer a problem for him to handle. He has accepted it as a way of life and has compensated for it through his ability to speechread. Larry's ability to adjust to the physical, emotional and mental traumas that he had was indeed rare. He is now managing his life well.

Appendix I

AUDIOLOGY: WHAT IS IT?

Audiology is a science that studies normal and abnormal hearing. Audiology was established as a science in 1945. Those who work as audiologists must have a minimum of a master's degree (approximately five to six years of university training) or a doctoral degree (approximately seven to eight years of university training). For educational or clinical purposes, a master's degree is fully adequate training. The doctoral degree is a research degree and does not provide the student with added clinical efficiency. Audiologists must be licensed in states that require it and hold the Certificate of Clinical Competence (CCC) given by the American Speech and Hearing Association.

The university or college education of audiologists includes physics, acoustics, instrumentation, anatomy, normal and abnormal speech development, normal and abnormal psychology, phonetics, language, linguistics, education and sociology.

Audiologists may teach at the college or university levels and may be involved in experimental research. They may direct a public or private school screening program or be an integral part of a private, public or government hearing clinic. Some audiologists also maintain a private practice.

Audiology is an outgrowth of medicine (otology) and special education (speech pathology). Audiologists are responsible for the knowledge of principles, methods and techniques of measuring, identifying, differentiating and evaluating hearing disorders and the necessary habilitation or rehabilitation of the hearing handicapped.

There is an ever growing need for the science of audiology in industry. It is hoped that it won't take years before this consultation is sought by large industries in need of such services. Audiologists are able to contribute significantly to the development of hearing conservation programs in industry. Audiologists can be vital in transferring employees from dangerously high noise levels to work environments that are far less threatening to hearing, ultimately protecting the hearing of numerous employees.

Appendix II

DRUGS THAT MAY BE HARMFUL TO HEARING

aconite
alcohol
aniline dyes
antipyrine
barbiturates
benzene
caffeine
camphor
carbon disulfide
carbon monoxide
Chenopodium
chloramphenicol
chloroform
chloroquinine
dihydrostreptomycin
ergot
gentamycin
hydrocyanic acid
iodine

iodoform
kanamycin
lead
mercury
morphine
neomycin
nitrobenzol
Novocain
Polybrene
quinidine
quinine
salicylates (aspirin)
salvarsan
streptomycin
sulfa drugs
tobacco
valerian
vancomycin
viomycin

Appendix III

WHERE TO WRITE FOR INFORMATION ON NOISE

Acoustical Society of America
A.I.P.
335 East 45th Street
New York, New York 10017

American Academy of Ophthalmology and Otolaryngology
15 Second Street, SW
Rochester, Minnesota 55901

American Mutual Insurance Alliance
20 North Wacker Drive
Chicago, Illinois 60606

American Society of Testing Materials
Noise Committee
1916 Race Street
Philadelphia, Pennsylvania 19103

American Speech and Hearing Association
Director of Public Information
9030 Old Georgetown Road
Washington, D.C. 20014

Citizens Against Noise
2729 West Lunt Avenue
Chicago, Illinois 60645

Citizens For A Quieter City, Inc.
Box 777
FDR Station
New York, New York 10022

Citizens League Against the Sonic Boom
19 Appleton Street
Cambridge, Massachusetts 02138

Consumer Protection and Environmental Health Services
U.S. Department of Health, Education and Welfare
Washington, D.C. 20204

Council on Environmental Quality
722 Jackson Place, NW
Washington, D.C. 20006

Environmental Defense Fund
1525 18th Street, NW
Washington, D.C. 20036
Phone: (202) 833-1484

Environmental Protection Agency Information Office
1626 K Street, NW
Washington, D.C. 20006

EPA REGIONAL NOISE REPRESENTATIVES:

    I. Mr. Al Hicks
       EPA—Region I
       JFK Building, Room 2113
       Boston, Massachusetts 02203
       Phone: (617) 223-5708

II. Mr. Emilio Escaladas
EPA—Region II
26 Federal Plaza
New York, New York 10007
Phone: (212) 264-2109

III. Mr. Patrick Anderson
EPA—Region III
Curtis Building
Sixth & Walnut Streets
Philadelphia, Pennsylvania 19106
Phone: (215) 597-9118

IV. Dr. Kent Williams
EPA—Region IV
1421 Peachtree Street, NE
Atlanta, Georgia 30309
Phone: (404) 526-5861

V. Mr. Horst Witschonke
EPA—Region V
230 South Dearborn
Chicago, Illinois 60604
Phone: (312) 353-7270

VI. Mr. Bob LaBreche
EPA—Region VI
1600 Patterson Street
Dallas, Texas 75201
Phone: (214) 749-7601

VII. Mr. Vincent Smith
EPA—Region VII
1735 Baltimore Street
Kansas City, Missouri 64108
Phone: (816) 374-3307

VIII. Mr. Robert Simmons
EPA—Region VIII
Suite 900, Lincoln Tower
Denver, Colorado 80203
Phone: (303) 837-2221

IX. Dr. Richard W. Procunier
EPA—Region IX
100 California Street
San Francisco, California 94111
Phone: (415) 556-4606

X. Ms. Deborah Yamamoto
EPA—Region X
1200 Sixth Avenue
Seattle, Washington 98101
Phone: (206) 442-1253

General Radio Corporation
300 Baker Avenue
Concord, Massachusetts 01742

Institute of Noise Control Engineering
Box 3206
Arlington Branch
Poughkeepsie, New York 12603

National Council on Noise Abatement
1625 K Street, NW
Washington, D.C. 20006

Occupational Safety and Health Administration
U.S. Department of Labor
Washington, D.C. 20210

Office of Noise Abatement
U.S. Department of Transportation
Washington, D.C. 20553

Society of Automotive Engineers
Noise Committee
485 Lexington Avenue
New York, New York 10017

Sound and Vibration Magazine
Circulation Manager
27101 East Oviatt Road
Bay Village, Ohio 44140

U.S. Government Printing Office
Superintendent of Documents
Washington, D.C. 20402

Washington Hearing & Speech Society
5255 Loughboro Road, NW
Washington, D.C. 20016
Phone: (202) 244-4420
         also
1934 Calvert Street, NW
Washington, D.C. 20009
Phone: (202) 265-7335

Washington Report, Editor
United Auto Workers
1125 15th Street, NW
Washington, D.C. 20009

Appendix IV

WHO TO CONTACT IF DISSATISFIED WITH HEARING AID PURCHASE OR SERVICE
(IF UNRESOLVED WITH DISPENSER)

Better Business Bureau (in your city)
Contact by phone or writing

Bureau of Consumer Affairs (in your city)
Department of Consumer Complaint and Protection
   re: Hearing Aid Dispensers (contact by phone)

State Board of Medical Examiners (in your state)
Department for Complaints with Hearing Aids
Contact by phone or write to the office in your state

National Hearing Aid Society
Board of Certification
20361 Middlebelt
Livonia, Michigan 48152
Phone: (313) 478-2610

Ombudsman
Public Affairs Department
Contact at any of your major radio or television broadcasting
   stations in your city.

Appendix V

WHERE TO WRITE FOR INFORMATION ON HEARING OR HEARING PROBLEMS

Alexander Graham Bell Association for the Deaf
1537 35th Street, NW
Washington, D.C. 20007

American Academy of Ophthalmology and Otolaryngology (AAOO)
15 Second Street, SW
Rochester, Minnesota 55901

American Council of Otolaryngology (ACO)
1100 17th Street, NW #406
Washington, D.C. 20036

American Speech and Hearing Association (ASHA)
9030 Old Georgetown Road
Washington, D.C. 20014

Better Hearing Institute
1430 K Street, NW
Suite 200
Washington, D.C. 20005

C.H.E.A.R.
International Foundation for Children's Hearing, Education and
  Research
871 McLean Avenue
Yonkers, New York 10704

Consumer Affairs Office in your city

Council of Organizations Serving The Deaf
Wilde Lake Village Green
Columbia, Maryland 21044

National Association of Speech and Hearing Action (NASHA)
814 Thayer Avenue #102
Silver Spring, Maryland 20910

National Association for The Deaf (NAD)
814 Thayer Avenue
Silver Spring, Maryland 20910

National Easter Seal Society for Crippled Children and Adults
2023 West Ogden Avenue
Chicago, Illinois 60612

The Volta Review
3417 Volta Place, NW
Washington, D.C. 20007

(NOTE: Most of these organizations offer publications that are
available upon request.)

Appendix VI

WHERE TO WRITE FOR INFORMATION ON PRODUCTS FOR TELEVISION AMPLIFICATION, TELEPHONE AMPLIFICATION, ALARM CLOCKS DESIGNED FOR HARD OF HEARING INDIVIDUALS, ETC.:

IN THE EAST WRITE

Hal-Hen Company
36-14 11th Street
Long Island, New York 11106

IN THE WEST WRITE

Televox Industries
6022 W. Pico Boulevard
Los Angeles, California 90035

Notes

1. Better Business Bureau, "Facts You Should Know About Hearing Aids" (Consumer Affairs Library, Better Business Bureau of Eastern Massachusetts, Inc., 1971).

2. Jerry Northern and Marion Downs, *Hearing in Children* (Williams and Wilkins Company, Baltimore, Maryland, 1974).

3. Retired Professional Action Group, *Paying Through the Ear* (Public Citizen, Inc., Philadelphia, 1973).

4. Helmer R. Myklebust, *The Psychology of Deafness,* second edition (Grune and Stratton, New York, 1964).

5. A. C. Kalischer, *Beethoven's Letters* (E. P. Dutton & Co., New York, 1926).

6. Helen Keller, *Helen Keller in Scotland* (Methuen and Co., London, 1933).

7. Aldous Huxley, *Words and Their Meaning* (Zeitlin Press, Los Angeles, 1940).

8. See note 6 above.

9. United States Department of Labor, "Noise: The Environmental Problem, A Guide to OSHA Standards" (Occupational Safety and Health Administration, Washington, D.C., 1972).

10. D. H. Eldridge and J. D. Miller, "Acceptable Noise Exposure—Damage Risk Criteria," *ASHA Reports No. 4: Noise As a Public Health Hazard* (The American Speech and Hearing Association, Washington, D.C., 1969).

11. *Guide for Conservation of Hearing in Noise,* A Supplement to the Transactions of the American Academy of Ophthalmology and Otolaryngology (Revised Edition, 1973).

175

12. Aram Glorig, "Thunderation," *Health & Science News* (January 1972).

13. William F. Rintelmann, "A Review of Research Concerning Rock and Roll Music and Noise-Induced Hearing Loss," *Maico Audiological Library Series* (vol. 8, report 7, 1970).

14. C. Speaks and D. A. Nelson, "TTS Following Exposure to Rock and Roll Music," *The Journal of The Acoustical Society of America* (vol. 45, 1969).

15. See note 13 above.

16. David M. Lipscomb, "Ear Damage from Exposure to Rock and Roll Music," *Archives of Otolaryngology* (vol. 90, 1969).

17. See note 16 above.

18. See note 1 above.

19. Alan J. Heffler, "Hearing Aids and Noise-Induced Hearing Loss," *Maico Audiological Library Series* (vol. 13, report 3, 1974).

20. Paul H. Ward, "Susceptibility to Auditory Fatigue," In *Contributions to Sensory Physiology, Vol. 3*, W. D. Neff, ed. (Academic Press, New York, 1968).

21. David M. Lipscomb, "Noise in the Environment: Recreational and Environmental Sounds," *Maico Audiological Library Series* (vol. 8, report 2, 1969).

22. C. T. Yarington, "Military Noise Induced Hearing Loss: Problem in Conservation Programs," *The Laryngoscope* (vol. 78, no. 4, 1968).

23. N. Olson, "Survey of Motor Vehicle Noise," *The Journal of the Acoustical Society of America* (vol. 52, no. 5, 1972).

24. J. E. Wesler, "Community Noise Survey of Medford," *The Journal of the Acoustical Society of America* (vol. 54, no. 4, 1973).

25. E. H. Nober, "Non-Auditory Effects of Noise," *Maico Audiological Library Series* (vol. 12, report 6, 1974).

26. P. Hurdle, S. R. Lane and W. C. Meecham, "Jet Aircraft Noise in Metropolitan Los Angeles Under Air Route Corridors," *The Journal of the Acoustical Society of America* (vol. 50, no. 1, 1971).

27. William Burns, *Noise and Man*, second edition (J. B. Lippincott Company, Philadelphia, 1973).

28. R. R. Coermann, *The Effects of Vibration and Noise on the Human Organism*, translated by G. L. Davies (Washington, D.C., Dept. of Commerce Publication 24679T, 1938).

29. Alexander Cohen, "Psychological Effects of Noise," *Noise As a Public Health Hazard,* W. D. Ward and J. E. Fricke, eds. (ASHA Reports 4, Washington, D.C., American Speech and Hearing Association, February 1969).

30. J. F. Corso, *The Effects of Noise on Human Behavior* (Report WADC No. 53-81 Wright Air Development Center, Wright-Patterson Air Force Base, Ohio, 1952).

31. Gerd Jansen, "Effects of Noise on Psychological State," *Noise As a Public Health Hazard,* W. D. Ward and J. E. Fricke, eds. (ASHA Reports No. 4, 1969).

32. H. J. Jerison and S. Wing, *Effects of Noise and Fatigue on a Complex Vigilance Task* (Report WADC, TR-57-14, Wright Development Center, Wright-Patterson Air Force Base, Ohio, 1957).

33. E. J. Murray, "Psychological Effects of Adverse Environmental Conditions and Their Implications for Adjusting in a Fallout Shelter," *National Academy of Sciences* (for OCDM) (Washington, D.C., Disaster Research Group, 1959).

34. Benjamin B. Weybrew, "Patterns of Psychophysiological Response to Military Stress," In *Psychological Stress,* Mortimer Appley and Richard Trumbell, eds. (Meredith Publishing Co., New York, 1961).

35. David M. Lipscomb, "Noise in the Environment: The Problem," *Maico Audiological Library Series* (vol. 8, report 1, 1969).

36. See note 9 above.

37. See note 28 above.

38. C. M. Sprock, W. F. Howard and F. C. Jacob, "Sound As a Deterrent to Rats and Mice," *Journal of Wildlife Management* (vol. 31, 1967).

39. W.D. Thompson and L.W. Sontag, "Behavioral Effects in the Offspring of Rats Subjected to Audiogenic Seizure During the Gestational Period," *Journal of Comparative and Physiological Psychology* (vol. 49, 1956).

40. G. Gonzalez, N. Miller and C. Istre, Jr., "Influence of Rocket Noise Upon Hearing in Guinea Pigs," *Aero Space Medicine* (vol. 41, 1970).

41. B. Zondek, "Effects of Auditory Stimuli on Female Reproductive Organs," *Transactions of the New England Obstetrical and Gynecological Society* (vol. 18, 1964).

42. H. Frings and F. Little, "Reactions of Honey Bees in the Hive to Simple Sounds," *Science* (vol. 125, 1957).

43. J. Bond, "Effects of Noise on the Physiology and Behavior of Farm Raised Animals," *Physiological Effects of Noise* (Plenum Press, New York, 1970).

44. United States Environmental Protection Agency, *Effects of Noise on Wildlife and Other Animals* (Washington, D.C., December 31, 1971).

45. See note 25 above.

46. A. Anthony and J. Harclerode, "Noise Stress in Laboratory Rodents II: Effects of Chronic Noise Exposure on Sexual Performance & Reproduction Function of Guinea Pigs," *The Journal of the Acoustical Society of America* (vol. 31, 1959).

47. A. Anthony, E. Ackerman and J. Lloyd, "Noise Stress in Laboratory Rodents I: Behavioral and Endocrine Response of Mice, Rats and Guinea Pigs," *The Journal of the Acoustical Society of America* (vol. 31, 1959).

48. M. Friedman, L. O. Byers and A. E. Brown, "Plasma Lipid Responses of Rats and Rabbits to an Auditory Stimulus," *American Journal of Physiology* (vol. 212, 1967).

49. See note 25 above.

50. See note 27 above.

51. See note 35 above.

52. See note 41 above.

53. See note 25 above.

54. See note 48 above.

55. See note 47 above.

56. See note 35 above.

57. See note 39 above.

58. See note 41 above.

59. L. B. Poche, C. W. Stockwell and H. W. Ades, "Cochlear Hair Cell Damage in Guinea Pigs After Exposure to Impulse Noise," *Journal of the Acoustical Society of America* (vol. 46, 1969).

60. See note 38 above.

61. See note 25 above.

62. Leonard Eisener, "Slants and Trends," *Noise Control Report* (October 2, 1972).

63. See note 11 above.

64. William G. Thomas, "Effects of Noise on Health and Hearing," Paper presented at the North Carolina Memorial Hospital Speech and Hearing Center, 1972.

65. See note 22 above.

66. Samuel Rosen et al., "Presbycusis Study of a Relatively Noise-Free Population in the Sudan," *Annals of Otology, Rhinology and Laryngology* (vol. 71, 1962).

67. Burton F. Jaffe, "Sudden Deafness," *Archives of Otolaryngology* (vol. 86, 1967).

68. Harold Schuknecht, "Mechanisms of Inner Ear Injury from Blows to the Head," *Annals of Otology, Rhinology and Laryngology* (vol. 78, no. 2, 1969).

69. Paul H. Ward, "The Histopathology of Auditory and Vestibular Disorders in Head Trauma," *Annals of Otology, Rhinology and Laryngology* (vol. 78, no. 2, 1969).

70. See note 69 above.

71. Harvey Kravitz et al., "The Cotton-Tipped Swab: A Major Cause of Ear Injury and Hearing Loss," *Clinical Pediatrics* (vol. 13, no. 11, 1974).

72. Edmund Fowler, "Subjective Head Noises," *Laryngoscope* (vol. 75, October 1965).

73. Egbert Huizing and Atze Spoor, "An Unusual Type of Tinnitus," *Archives of Otolaryngology* (vol. 98, 1973).

74. Jerome Alpiner, "Some Aspects of Tinnitus Aurium as Related to Hearing Impairment," *Maico Audiological Library Series* (vol. 5, report 1, 1966).

75. See note 72 above.

76. J.T. Graham and H.A. Newby, "Tinnitus Aurium," *Archives of Otolaryngology* (vol. 75, 1962).

77. M. Friedman et al., "Effect of Unsaturated Fats Upon Lipemia and Conjunctival Circulation: A Study of Coronary-Prone (Pattern A) Men," *Journal of the American Medical Association* (vol. 193, 1965).

78. C.B. Taylor et al., "Atherosclerosis in Rhesus Monkeys," *Archives of Pathology* (vol. 76, 1963).

79. M. C. Armstrong et al., "Regression of Coronary Atheromatosis in Rhesus Monkeys," *Circulation Research* (vol. 27, 1970).

80. C. Tucker et al., "Regression of Cholesterol-Induced Atherosclerotic Lesions in Rhesus," *Circulation* (supplement 2, vol. 63, 1971).

81. M. Bierenbaum et al., "The V-Year Experience of Modified Fat Diets on Young Men with Coronary Heart Diseases," *Circulation* (vol. 42, 1970).

82. J. B. Hannab, "Civilization, Race and Coronary Atheroma with Particular Reference to its Severity in Africans," *Central African Journal of Medicine* (vol. 4, 1958).

83. A. P. Walker et al., "Glucose and Fat Tolerance in Bantu Children," *The Lancet* (July 4, 1970).

84. See note 66 above.

85. W. Enos, R. H. Holmes and J. Boyer, "Coronary Disease Among United States Soldiers Killed in Action in Korea," *Journal of the American Medical Association* (vol. 152, July 18, 1953).

86. Samuel Rosen and Pekka Olin, "Hearing Loss and Coronary Heart Disease," *Archives of Otolaryngology* (vol. 82, September 1965).

87. See note 86 above.

88. Samuel Rosen, P. Olin and Helen V. Rosen, "Dietary Prevention of Hearing Loss," *Acta Otolaryngologica* (vol. 70, 1970).

89. Samuel Rosen et al., "Relation of Hearing Loss to Cardiovascular Disease," *Transactions of the American Academy of Opthalmology and Otolaryngology* (vol. 68, 1964).

90. Michael M. Paparella, *Biochemical Mechanisms in Hearing and Deafness* (Charles C Thomas, Springfield, Illinois, 1970).

91. Stephen V. Prescod, "Effects of Tobacco Smoking on the Auditory System," *Maico Audiological Library Series* (vol. 14, report 9, 1976).

92. Public Health Service, "Smoking and Health," (PHS Publication No. 1103, 1964, pages 5-30).

93. O. Paul et al., "Study of Coronary Heart Disease," *Circulation* (vol. 28, 1963).

94. S. Bellet et al., "Response of Free Fatty Acid to Coffee and Caffeine," *Metabolism* (vol. 17, 1968).

95. Abraham Shulman, "The Pill, Hearing and Balance," *Highlights* (Quarterly Bulletin: New York League for the Hard of Hearing, 1974).

96. See note 90 above.

97. "A Collection of Shared Letters," *Zenith Professional and Educational Services* (Zenith Hearing Instrument Corporation, vol. 5, no. 1, May 1974).

98. Gerald English, Jerry Northern and Thomas J. Fria, "Chronic Otitis Media As a Cause of Sensorineural Hearing Loss," *Archives of Otolaryngology* (vol. 98, July 1973).

99. Marcus Diamant and Bertel Diamant, "Abuse and Timing of Use of Antibiotics in Acute Otitis Media," *Archives of Otolaryngology* (vol. 100, September 1974).

100. See note 98 above.

101. D. L. Cowan and M. J. K. M. Brown, "Seromucinous Otitis Media and Its Sequelae (A Retrospective Study of 242 Children)," *Journal of Laryngology and Otology* (vol. 88, no. 12, 1974).

102. Alaa El Seifi, "Myringoplasty (Repair of Total or Subtotal Drum Perforations)," *Journal of Laryngology and Otology* (vol. 88, no. 8, 1974).

103. Tos Mirko, "Tympanoplasty and Age," *Archives of Otolaryngology* (vol. 96, 1972).

104. Karl H. Siedentop, Lee R. Hamilton and Stan B. Osenar, "Predictability of Tympanoplasty Results," *Archives of Otolaryngology* (vol. 95, 1972).

105. J. D. K. Dawes and A. R. Curry, "Types of Stapedectomy Failure and Prognosis of Revision of Operations," *Journal of Laryngology and Otology* (vol. 88, no. 3, 1974).

106. Harold Ludman and Henry Grant, "The Case Against Bilateral Stapedectomy, and the Problems of Post-Operative Follow-Up from the King's College Hospital Series," *Journal of Laryngology and Otology* (vol. 87, no. 9, 1973).

107. N. Shah, "Revision Stapedectomy for Late Conductive Deafness," *Journal of Laryngology and Otology* (vol. 88, 1974).

108. John Lindsay, "Histopathology of Otosclerosis," *Archives of Otolaryngology* (vol. 97, 1973).

109. Richard Pearson, Leonard Kurland and D. Thane R. Cody, "Incidence of Diagnosed Clinical Otosclerosis," *Archives of Otolaryngology* (vol. 99, 1974).

110. Hallowell Davis and Richard Silverman, *Hearing and Deafness*, third edition (Holt, Rinehart and Winston, Inc., New York, 1970).

111. M. Spencer Harrison and Lionel Naftalin, *Meniere's Disease* (Charles C Thomas, Springfield, Illinois, 1970).

112. Better Business Bureau, "Facts About Hearing Aids" (Consumer Information Series, Council of Better Business Bureaus, Inc., 1973).

113. See note 19 above.

114. See note 1 above.

115. See note 3 above.

116. See note 3 above.

117. *ASHA,* a journal of the American Speech and Hearing Association (vol. 17, no. 1, January 1975), p. 33.

118. See note 3 above.

119. "Health and Medicine," *Consumer Reports* (May 1971), p. 310.

120. See note 19 above.

121. Geary McCandless and David Miller, "Loudness Discomfort and Hearing Aids," *National Hearing Aid Journal* (vol. 7, 1972).

122. Janet Jeffers and Margaret Barley, *Speechreading (Lipreading)* (Charles C Thomas, Springfield, Illinois, 1974).

Index

A

acupuncture, as cure, 71, 72 148-151
acute otitis media, treatment of, 74, 75
adults, hearing loss in, effects of, 8-11
aged. See *elderly.*
air traffic, noise and, 41-43
aircraft, noise and, 41-43
alcohol, hearing loss and, 65, 108
antibiotics, hearing loss and, 68
appliances, for hard of hearing, 173
aspirin, hearing loss and, 66
    tinnitus and, 152
audiogram, description of, 19
    example of, 20
    hearing loss and, 21, 22
audiologists, education of, 159
    need for, 86
audiology, definition of, 159, 160
automobiles, noise and, 40

B

bathing, earwax and, 106
batteries, for hearing aids, 129-131
Beethoven, Ludwig van, 13, 14
blindness, orientation and, 15, 16
bones, of ear, 22, 23

C

caffeine, hearing loss and, 66
cells, hair, damage to, 24
cerumen, characteristics of, 58
    production of, 57, 58
    removal of, 58, 59, 106
    showering and, 106
children, deaf, schooling of, 117, 118
    deafness and, 114-116
    hearing aids and, 113, 114
    hearing loss in, effects of, 6-8
        incidence of, 2, 3, 38

V

vitamins, as cure, 69-70
vocabulary, hearing loss
    and, 7
vowels, frequency of, 27, 28
    speech and, 27, 28

W

wages, loss of, hearing loss and,
    47, 48
whiskey. See *alcohol.*
workers, industrial, hearing loss
    in, 2, 3
        hearing problems and,
            39, 48, 49